The Anatomy of Pilates

Paul Massey

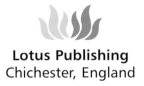

Lotus Publishing
Chichester, England

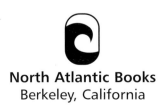

North Atlantic Books
Berkeley, California

First published in 2009 by
Lotus Publishing
Apple Tree Cottage, Inlands Road, Nutbourne, PO18 8RJ and
North Atlantic Books
P O Box 12327
Berkeley, California 94712

Anatomical Drawings Amanda Williams, Pascale Pollier, Emily Evans and Inga Borg
Text Design and Line Drawings Wendy Craig
Cover Design Jim Wilkie
Printed and Bound in the UK by Scotprint

Disclaimer

This book is not meant as a substitute for medical advice. If you have any medical condition or if you experience pain or discomfort with the exercises contained within this book, then you must stop immediately and consult a qualified medical practitioner. Both the Publisher and the Author accept no responsibility for any consequences of the advice given if medical advice is not sought and followed before beginning a new exercise programme.

The Anatomy of Pilates is sponsored by the Society for the Study of Native Arts and Sciences, a nonprofit educational corporation whose goals are to develop an educational and crosscultural perspective linking various scientific, social, and artistic fields; to nurture a holistic view of arts, sciences, humanities, and healing; and to publish and distribute literature on the relationship of mind, body, and nature.

British Library Cataloguing in Publication Data
A CIP record for this book is available from the British Library
ISBN 978 1 905367 13 9 (Lotus Publishing)
ISBN 978 1 55643 780 9 (North Atlantic Books)

Library of Congress Cataloging-in-Publication Data

Massey, Paul, MCSP.
  The anatomy of pilates / Paul Massey.
      p. ; cm.
  ISBN 978-1-905367-13-9 (Lotus Publishing) -- ISBN 978-1-55643-780-9 (North Atlantic Books)
  1. Pilates method. 2. Musculoskeletal system--Anatomy. I. Title.
  [DNLM: 1. Exercise Movement Techniques--methods. 2. Musculoskeletal System--anatomy & histology. 3. Movement--physiology. 4. Posture--physiology. WB 541 M416a 2009]
  RA781.4.M37 2009
  613.7'192--dc22
                                        2008049026

Contents

Introduction

Born in 1880 in Munchengladbach, near Düsseldorf, Germany, Joseph Pilates was a skinny, sickly child, suffering from rickets, asthma and rheumatic fever.

He worked to develop an exercise regime that might improve his own health, and so involved himself in a number of physical activities to improve his body form. These activities included boxing, gymnastics, skiing and self-defence, as he developed his muscular definition through physical activity. He even posed for anatomy charts as he developed his muscular profile.

Pilates moved to England in 1912, training further as a boxer and self-defence instructor. But in 1914 the First World War broke out, and along with other German nationals he was put into internment camps in Lancaster and then the Isle of Man. During this time he taught physical training to other inmates of the camps and developed rehabilitation programmes for those injured during the War.

After the War in 1919, Pilates returned to Germany to train the Hamburg Military Police in self-defence and physical fitness. It was at this time that he worked with Rudolph Laban, a movement analyst who worked with dancers. Laban worked on establishing training programmes for the fitness industry, collaborating with Pilates and utilizing his ideas. Pilates was approached to work with the German army but, unhappy at this prospect, decided to leave for America.

On the journey to America in 1926, the 45-year-old Pilates met his wife-to-be, Clara, and together they established a studio on Eighth Avenue, New York, in the same building as several dance studios. This location, being in close proximity to the dance world, was pivotal to how the Pilates exercise regime came to be closely associated with the conditioning, rehabilitation from injury and training of many dancers.

At this point in his life, Pilates developed his own exercise training method called CONTROLOGY. Training in his method was by apprenticeship and, once qualified, the apprentices would go on to open their own schools and develop the method, introducing their own ideas and approaches.

Joseph Pilates' greatest legacy remains his classic exercises. Many Pilates schools teach and progress them differently, with the end product being an evolving method. This book illustrates the classical exercise programme in detail, with breathing, movement and aims applied throughout.

The Pilates Method Alliance®, the professional association and awarding body dedicated to the teachings of Joseph Pilates, stated that:

"Pilates exercise focuses on postural symmetry, breath control, abdominal strength, spine, pelvis and shoulder stabilization, muscle flexibility, joint mobility and strengthening through the complete range of motion of all joints instead of isolating muscle groups, the whole body is trained, integrating the upper and lower extremities with the trunk."

The Pilates Method Alliance® further stated that:

"Today it is acceptable to apply the principles of Pilates to all forms of movement and exercise, and sport and daily life activities as Joseph intended."

As mentioned, the Pilates Method has progressed to a physical and mental conditioning exercise regime, using clearly defined movement patterns. The emphasis is on quality of movement and not quantity/volume of repetitions.

The movements or exercises undertaken follow a defined, precise sequence that incorporates a particular breathing pattern linked to the controlled exercise.

The complete mat programme used in this book allows every muscle group to be worked, with attention to the sequence of the stabilizing muscles then the mobilizing muscles as the ability to undertake the exercise progresses. The Principle of Pilates movement applies throughout each of the exercises.

Chapter

1

Introduction
to the
Pilates Method

Principles of the Pilates Method

Concepts and Elements Used in the Pilates Method

Breathing

The Anatomy of Pilates

Pilates is an exercise regime that can be described as a unique method of body conditioning, combining muscle strengthening and flexibility with a breathing method that works to establish coordination between the trunk, scapulae and pelvis during movement. Furthermore, it acts as a tool to restore muscle balance to the musculo-skeletal system during movement.

Principles of the Pilates Method

Joseph Pilates claimed that his method had both a philosophical and theoretical foundation, being more than just a collection of exercises based on the mat, but a method that developed over a number of years, based on use and observation.

The main element of the Pilates method is considered to be a mind–body conditioning programme, which enables the body to move with less effort, allowing a flowing and balanced movement. The method uses the individual's own body to its greatest advantage, utilising its own strength, muscle flexibility and coordination, and requires that the individual pay attention to his or her body throughout the exercise.

In order to achieve this mind–body connection, the following principles are considered to be the main components of all mat work exercises.

1. Control

For any training in an exercise technique, there needs to be a level of awareness that is progressive to the method, to help correct alignment and encourage precision/flowing movement. This ability to control movement develops through every aspect of the movement, and skill levels increase as the complexity of the movement sequence increases. Control or awareness needs to be achieved throughout every exercise. Being aware of the position of all your body parts, by maintaining a neutral spine position and through the use of the deep stabilizer muscles, enhances and maintains the correct alignment.

It is not about the intensity of the movement, but rather the ability to move with quality, by the activation of the correct muscles in the right sequence for that exercise/movement. When undertaking Pilates exercises, good technique brings about safe, effective results.

2. Centre

Focus on the specific muscles that control the core/key areas, which enable the rest of the body to function efficiently.

Activate the tonic holding muscles in the required static position. There needs to be an ability to hold the required stabilizer(s) at a low level for periods of time.

All the actions of the exercises need to take place from a stable core and through correct activation of the powerhouse (see page 12).

3. Concentration

This involves the important mind–body connection. Focusing on the muscle(s) as you practise will enhance your ability to perform the movement correctly. You need to be constantly aware of your whole body throughout each exercise.

The ability to undertake the exercise and skill are closely linked. You must always intend to perform the exercise in the correct way. This is enhanced by knowing the exercise objectives, from the start to the finish.

Positional sense, or proprioception, is the normal awareness of the joint–body position or motion, generated by sensory feedback. This skill can be developed, and needs to be continually challenged in order to improve. There should be a balanced state between movement and a movement pattern, which builds into a functional movement. Feel the movement – don't just execute it.

4. Precision

Concentrate on the right movement each time you undertake the exercise. The correct procedure each time will allow for correct progression. Do not rely on pure strength to complete the exercise but be sensitive to the quality needed to undertake it.

5. Flowing movements

Quality of movement is linked closely with control. There should be no stiffness or jerkiness, and movement should be smooth and continuous.

Quality is a result of working smarter rather than harder, and enhances the good movement pattern that develops throughout the Pilates programme. *"There is no such thing as bad exercise, just exercise done badly."*

Encourage the use of muscle groups instead of isolated muscle action. Coordination or sequence of movement is essential. Initially perform each exercise slowly, and then increase the speed; further progression can be achieved by changing direction and speed during the exercise, and the use of more than one joint (upper or lower limb) at a time. Movement efficiency is a balance between muscle relaxation and muscle contraction; correct balance allows good quality movement, which is necessary during a Pilates exercise.

6. Breathing

Breathing is an automatic, necessary activity, and as such influences the body's activities. Focusing on breathing promotes attention and awareness. Emphasise breathing with the movement and, importantly, not holding your breath.

Breathing can be seen as a link between physical activity and the inside–outside of the body. A correct breathing pattern increases awareness, thoracic (trunk) control, and use of the lower ribs. It also enhances the connection between the pelvic floor and the diaphragm.

Lateral costal breathing, wide and full out through the ribs, requires breathing in on the point of effort, and out on the return of exhalation.

If you are doing something that tightens your body, use the motion to squeeze air out of your lungs and inhale when you straighten up. This forced technique was seen by Joseph Pilates as the key to full inhalation during each exercise. (There is more about breathing later on page 15.)

7. Alignment

Correct alignment in any exercise needs to be in the correct posture, working primarily from a neutral position of the spine.

8. Coordination

Movement that is coordinated needs to be learnt; this is achieved by correct repetition of an exercise, and provides a good foundation for advancement.

9. Stamina

Challenging the control and correct procedure of each exercise will allow development of the stamina needed to undertake the exercises. Stamina can be seen as the improvement of strength and challenge to the muscles used in the exercise, allowing for repetitive quality movements.

10. Lengthening

This can be seen as the development of flexibility of the muscles used in the exercise. Muscles need to be able to maintain length to allow for correct movement.

The Anatomy of Pilates

Concepts and Elements Used in the Pilates Method

Powerhouse
The powerhouse is formed of a number of muscles around the lumbar spine, between the bottom of the ribs and the line across the hips. The Pilates Method focuses on specific muscles to enhance this powerhouse concept: rectus abdominis, the obliques, multifidus, transversus abdominis, the pelvic floor, the diaphragm, gluteal group and the psoas. These are the main stabilizer muscles of the trunk/lower limbs.

The powerhouse is worked in all Pilates exercises, as it achieves a stable base from which to work, enhances coordination between core areas, and supports the spine during movement.

The secondary powerhouse is around the shoulder girdle. Its function is to stabilize and enhance quality movement around the upper limb during exercise.

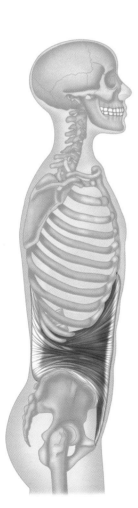

Muscles involved include the lower trapezius, serratus anterior, latissimus dorsi, pectorals and deep neck flexors.

Transversus abdominis is the main powerhouse muscle; it is the deepest, and covers the abdomen. This muscle needs to be activated at the start of all Pilates exercises, and continually engaged throughout.

How to Locate Transversus Abdominis
Place your fingers just inside your hip bones. While maintaining a neutral spine (no movement in the small of your back), breathe out, draw up the muscles of the pelvic floor, and hollow in the abdominals (the area below your belly button). Ensure you work at a low intensity.

You should feel your fingers draw down and not push up. (If you feel them push up, you are working too hard, and so using your oblique abdominal muscles.) You need to be able to hold this position with no pelvic tilt or movement. Stability muscles such as transversus abdominis need only work at less than 30 per cent of their full-effort maximum voluntary contraction (MVC – a measure of strength).

Figure 1.1: Transversus abdominis.

Verbal Cues to Help Locate Transversus Abdominis

Scoop the stomach, navel to spine. Pull in your stomach and your navel. Zip up and hollow. Keep your abdomen drawn in. This activation is undertaken in a neutral spine position.*

Individuals need to work from their own base lines; it is a changeable position during each exercise, but needs to be maintained when activating the deep stabilizing abdominal muscles, and not moved with the contraction.

Box

Draw an imaginary line connecting your two shoulders to each other, and your two hip bones to each other, and then a vertical line connecting them, so that a rectangle is drawn on your trunk.

If this box is superimposed on your body, it will help you keep your hips square and away from your ribs, the base of your spine positioned in relation to the mat, and your shoulders in alignment and away from your ears while you move. This will aid trunk–body alignment and symmetry, and hence the activation of your powerhouse.

Moving Without Tension

Undertaking the Pilates exercises does not mean tightening up muscles in order to achieve the exercise. You need to think through the principles and their application to achieve your goal. Tensing up, holding your breath, and pushing to strain will only lead to jarring movement, poor quality and a possible inability to move to the end goal of the exercise or end position.

The exercises do need strength and coordination in order to flow and connect; an element of relaxation into the movement is also required. You need to think and identify from where the movement will be required to come, work within your ability, and then build to reach your end goal of a quality, controlled, flowing movement.

Guidelines to good exercise

1. Work within your ability.
2. Build from the centre into the arms and legs (need for a strong centre: powerhouse).
3. Maintain a correct breathing pattern.
4. Don't tense in order to move.

*The position of the neutral spine during exercise is one that is individual, and defined as a balanced state between normal tissue length in the spine and the muscles (front to back) of the trunk.

No Pain, No Gain

This statement has no place in a Pilates programme. If you find you are building up excessive tension in an area during the exercise, stop, review the instructions for that exercise, and continue.

If pain or tension does return, stop that exercise and leave it out of your programme. Each of the Pilates exercises can be broken down into small components, so note where the problem occurs, and build the movement up to the point where you have sufficient strength or length to continue.

Area of Discomfort	Possible Cause
Lower back	Losing the contraction of the powerhouse. Working with your extremities beyond your capability. (Work from the trunk out into your arms and legs.)
Knee	Incorrect foot or leg positioning. Weak thigh muscles around the joint. Altered muscle alignment to the lower limb.
Hip	Loss of neutral spine. Muscle imbalance around the pelvis.
Neck	Muscle weakness around the neck. Loss of coordination between the scapular base and neck. Weak scapular stabilization.

Solution

1. Work with the Pilates principle during the exercise.
2. Work from the centre outward.
3. Listen to your body and avoid excessive tension.

Breathing

Breathing is important for exercise, and correct breathing is a foundation of all Pilates exercises. Joseph Pilates endorsed active inhalation and exhalation from the viewpoint of cleansing the lungs, which was encouraged in all of the classic mat exercises; current research indicates a link between breathing and trunk stability.

Breathing Pattern

Inhalation
During inhalation, the volume of the thoracic cavity is increased, drawing in air through the nose/mouth into the lungs. The process starts with the contraction of the diaphragm, which initially lowers into the abdominal cavity, increasing the volume of the thoracic cavity. Expansion of the rib cage is initiated by the diaphragm. Contraction and the activation of the external intercostal muscles enhance the process.

Exhalation
During exhalation, the diaphragm and muscles involved in inhalation relax, the diaphragm ascends, and the rib cage drops. This is enhanced by the contraction of the internal intercostal muscles and the recoil of the lung tissue/thoracic cavity.

Forced exhalation is achieved by contraction of the abdominal (external obliques) and other muscles associated with breathing.

Each Pilates exercise has a specific breathing pattern. Breathing is a skill, and coordination of the breathing and the exercise needs to be practised.

A general teaching point is to use the exhalation phase of the breathing pattern on the work (effort) part of the exercise (usually involving spinal flexion), and the inhalation phase on the return part of the exercise (usually involving spinal extension).

Breathing should occur naturally, so avoid forced active exhalation. (As stated by Joseph Pilates in his initial works, but it has been found that this pattern can lead to early recruitment and over-recruitment of the external obliques, which may alter spinal stability.)

The correct breathing pattern for Pilates exercises is lateral costal breathing, drawing in long, deep breaths to expand the rib cage to its fullest capacity, followed by full (but not forced) exhalation to deflate the lungs.

The muscles of respiration do not work in isolation but are connected to the ribs and spine and also play a large role in postural control.

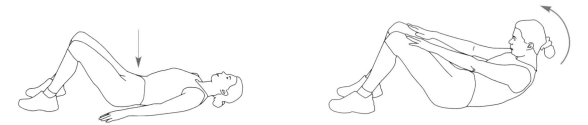

Figure 1.2: The curl-up. See arrows, showing the work (effort) phase and return phase of the exercise.

Muscle Involved in Respiration

1.Diaphragm
The diaphragm is the main inspiratory muscle. Contraction of the muscle causes the dome of the diaphragm to descend, so enlarging the dimension of the thorax in all directions (cranially, caudally and sideward).

The diaphragm contributes to spinal stability via an increase in intra-abdominal pressure, and with transversus abdominis, continually works to control trunk movement and enhance the breathing pattern during movement, particularly involving the extremities.

2. Intercostals
These small muscles are responsible for the lateral expansion of the chest and stabilization of the ribs during inspiration. They have a close anatomical connection with the internal and external oblique muscles, a further link to the active inspiration.

3. Abdominal muscles
This is the main muscle group involved in forced expiration. These muscles alter the intra-abdominal pressure to assist the emptying of the lungs and transmit the pressure generated by the diaphragm.

Note: intra-abdominal pressure is the pressure created in the trunk, in the closed cylinder of the diaphragm, pelvic floor and abdominal wall. Greater pressure adds stability to the trunk and pelvis. Use of an increased intra-abdominal pressure to maintain stability is not actively recommended due to its detrimental effect on circulation and blood pressure, and it has a limited role.

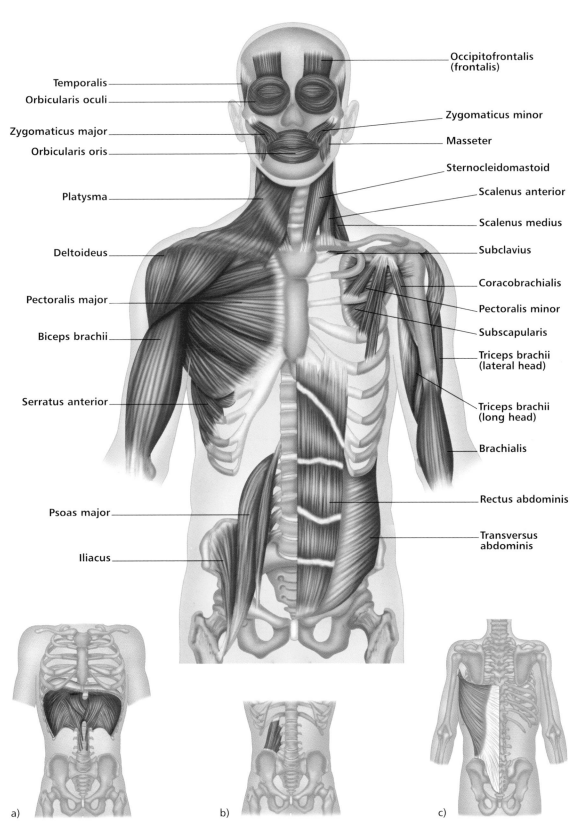

Figure 1.3: The upper body, anterior view, showing the key muscles of respiration, including the diaphragm (a), quadratus lumborum (b), and latissimus dorsi (c, posterior view).

The Anatomy of Pilates

4. Pelvic floor muscles
This is a collective group of muscles and soft tissue that makes up the base of the abdominal cavity. These have a role in the maintenance of the intra-abdominal pressure and transference of the stability created by the respiratory process.

Other muscle groups activated during correct breathing activation work with the main respiratory muscles but become activated when the exercise becomes demanding, or when there is a change in position during the exercise. They are needed to stabilize parts of the body to enhance the respiratory action.

- The scalene muscles aid in deep inspiration by fixing the 1st and 2nd ribs, and maintain them during expiration against the contraction of the abdominal muscles.
- Sternocleidomastoid elevates the sternum and increases the forward and backward dimension of the chest during moderate to deep inspiration if the cervical spine is held stable.
- Serratus anterior assists in inspiration to laterally expand the rib cage, if the scapulae are stabilized.
- The pectorals act in forced inspiration to raise the ribs; the scapulae need to be stabilized by trapezius and serratus anterior to prevent scapular winging.
- Latissimus dorsi is involved in forced inspiration and expiration.
- Erector spinae helps in respiration by extending the thoracic spine and raising the rib cage.
- Quadratus lumborum stabilizes the 12th rib to prevent elevation during respiration.

Ideal Breathing Pattern
There are a number of factors that need to be taken into consideration when assessing the breathing pattern:

1. Balance between the amount and quality of movement taking place in the different areas of the thorax: apical (at the apex), abdominal and lateral costal.

2. Which muscles are in use: diaphragm, abdominals or accessory muscles of breathing.

3. Timing/rhythm of breathing: an even time spent on inhalation and exhalation; there is also a need for short pauses between phases.

4. Background posture.

While in a relaxed state, inhale through your nose, breathing wide and full into your ribs, ensuring you don't allow the apical area of the chest to rise. Note the air entering the base of the lung. Movement is into the side of the ribs.

As you breathe in, slowly and gently engage your lower abdominal muscles and transversus abdominis. Draw in this lower abdominal area slightly when engaging tranversus abdominis, so that you feel the area flatten. Exhalation is relaxed.

Points for consideration in the abdominals during breathing:

- need for contraction of transversus abdominis
- no bulging of the lower abdominal area, which may indicate over-activity in the internal obliques
- inability to relax the abdominals between breathing cycles
- out breath – sternum softening, rib cage closing down
- in breath – expansion of the rib cage, relaxed shoulder girdle

Inefficient Breathing Pattern
1. Dominance of apical breathing. Contributing factors:

- breathing undertaken by dominance of the accessory muscles of inspiration
- excessive movement dominance of the upper ribs
- loss of ideal head posture (towards forward head posture)
- increased thoracic kyphosis
- vertical shoulder girdle movement due to muscle imbalance, tight scalenes, suprascapular muscles and reduced activation of serratus anterior

2. Insufficient lateral costal breathing due to restricted lateral and/or posterior rib cage expansion.

3. Dominance of abdominal breathing due to over-activity of the superficial abdominal muscle (external oblique muscles have been shown to fix or tighten in length due to the presence of chronic low back pain, which leads to alteration in the muscle activation pattern of inhalation).

4. Abnormal movement pattern. Changes in movement pattern may occur due to thoracic–lumbar flexion resulting from increased activity in external obliques and rectus abdominis. Also, as a result of a depressed rib cage due to over-activation of the external obliques muscles.

5. Musculo-skeletal considerations:

- over-developed thoraco-lumbar erector spinae
- reduced thoraco-lumbar movement
- increased activation of the external obliques and rectus abdominis
- inability to breathe diaphragmatically

Factors to Ensure an Ideal Breathing Pattern

1. Client relaxation

Reduce	Techniques
Fear and anxiety	Sighing
Breath holding	Long exhalation phase
Breathlessness	Slow and deep rhythm
Tension in accessory muscles	Conscious release of muscle tension due to correct positioning

2. Maintenance of ideal background postural alignment
Correct postural alignment will allow for the correct muscle length and tension to be maintained, and hence the ability to contract when required, when moving during the exercise.

3. Pattern appropriate to the exercise
The breathing pattern needs to flow in a correct sequence, inhalation and exhalation. Altered timing in either cycle or holding your breath leads to abnormal breathing patterns.

4. Skeletal muscle balance
Changes in skeletal muscle balance influencing the breathing cycle lead to abnormal breathing patterns. Muscle imbalances that may be present include:

- overactive erector spinae, scalenes and trapezius
- underactive serratus anterior and abdominals
- kyphotic posture (restriction in the rib cage and thoracic spine)

Chapter

2

Posture and Movement Assessment

The Anatomy of Pilates

Posture

Posture is the position in which you hold your body upright against gravity while standing, sitting or lying down. Good posture involves training your body to stand, walk, sit and lie in positions where the least strain is placed on supporting muscles and ligaments during movement or weight-bearing activities. Proper posture includes keeping the bones and joints in the correct alignment so that muscles are being used properly, which helps to prevent the spine from becoming fixed in abnormal positions.

Assessment Tool

Postural assessment is crucial as a starting point to create a comprehensive Pilates programme. The assessment process can take one of two approaches:

1. Static: indicating muscle imbalance or changes in muscle length (long, weak, short or tight). Static posture will indicate possible areas to note, and so alter movement quality and ability to undertake the exercise.

2. Dynamic: through movement testing in specific activities, dynamic exercise will illustrate any incorrect movement pattern, so helping to determine the appropriate Pilates exercises to undertake.

Factors influencing posture include:

- inherited conditions, i.e. your genetic make-up
- habitual positions you undertake during your occupation or during repetitive movements, or postural alignment changes in response to the nature of the activity
- pathology, due to the presence of a disease
- trauma, resulting in damage to tissue or bones
- altered muscle balance, i.e. changes in the interplay between different muscles or muscle groups

Posture Types

Lordotic Posture (Lordosis)

This is indicated by an exaggeration of the lumbar curve. Features include:

- anterior tilt of the pelvis
- lengthened/weak rectus abdominis and external obliques
- lengthened, weak or underactive gluteus maximus and medius
- hamstrings which are somewhat elongated but may or may not be weak (Kendall & McCreary, 1983)
- overactive and tight hamstrings

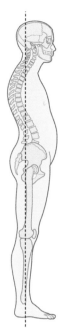

- flexed hip position
- short and strong low back and hip flexor muscles
- tight adductors due to flexed hip position

Recommendations to manage a lordotic posture:

- strengthen and shorten abdominal muscles (rectus abdominis, external obliques)
- enhance flexibility of the back extensors (multifidus and erector spinae)
- enhance flexibility of the hip flexors and adductors
- build flexibility into the hamstrings

Suggested exercises:

Bridge, Hamstring Stretch, Curl-up, Roll-up

Figure 2.1: Lordotic posture.
Note the exaggerated lumbar curve.

Flat Back Posture
Indicated by a reduced lumbar curve. Features include:

- weak neck flexors (head forward)
- thoracic forward curve (upper part)
- reduced lumbar curve
- posterior pelvis tilt
- tight or short rectus abdominis, frequently strong
- short and strong hamstrings
- lengthened and weak hip flexors
- knee hyperextended, or may be slightly flexed

Recommendations to manage a flat back posture:

- lengthen hamstrings
- strengthen or shorten hip flexors
- lengthen rectus abdominis

Suggested exercises:

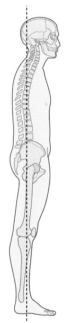

Figure 2.2: Flat back posture.
Note the reduced lumbar curve.

Curl-up, Single Leg Stretch, Swimming, Roll-up

The Anatomy of Pilates

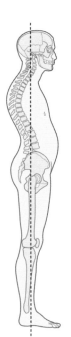

Kyphotic Posture (Kyphosis)
Indicated by an exaggerated curvature in the thoracic spine. Features include:

- head or chin poking forward
- cervical spine in hyperextension
- upper trapezius overactive or shortened
- scapulae abducted from the trunk
- thoracic spine flexed
- thoracic extensors lengthened
- pectoralis muscles shortened or tight
- rectus abdominis tight
- lower trapezius and serratus anterior lengthened or inactive
- posterior deltoid lengthened

Figure 2.3: Kyphotic posture. Note the exaggerated curvature in the thoracic spine.

Recommendations to manage a kyphotic posture:

- improve the alignment of head posture
- strengthen lower and middle trapezius, rhomboids and posterior deltoid
- improve strength around the shoulder girdle
- improve pelvic alignment
- improve flexibility of the thoracic spine
- improve control of scapular retraction and depression
- stretch pectoral muscles
- passive back extensions

Suggested exercises:

Double Leg Circles, Spine Twist, Roll-up, Swan Dive

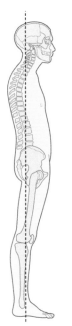

Figure 2.4: Sway back posture. Note the hips pushed forward.

Sway Back Posture
Indicated by the hips pushed forward and anterior tilt of the pelvis. The lordosis changes shape from an even curve to a deeper, shorter curve. The thoracic kyphosis is longer and may extend into the lumbar spine. Features include:

- head poking forward
- weak neck flexors
- long lower thoracic spine, leaning backward (posterior sway)
- slightly kyphotic stance
- weak or lengthened thoracic extensors
- lumbar spine flexed and flattened
- pelvis level, but hips pushed forward
- posterior tilt
- weak and lengthened hip flexors; hips are effectively extended so that the body 'hangs' on the hip ligaments
- gluteals shortened or weakened
- tensor fascia latae tight
- knees hyperextended
- hamstrings short and strong
- external obliques lengthened, internal obliques unchanged or shortened

Recommendations to manage a sway back posture:

- improve standing postural alignment
- lengthen the spine
- strengthen deep neck flexors
- strengthen trapezius
- lengthen hamstrings
- strengthen erector spinae
- lengthen pectorals and anterior deltoid (if shoulders protracted, although that is not always associated with this postural type)
- shorten or strengthen hip flexors

Suggested exercises:

Curl-up, Leg Pull Back, Spine Stretch Forward, Spine Twist

The Anatomy of Pilates

Postural Assessment

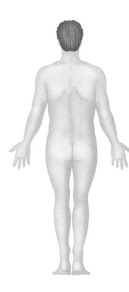

Figure 2.5: Standing view of the body, posterior view.

Head	Neutral	Side bent R/L	Rotated R/L
Shoulders	Level	Asymmetrical	
Scapular position	Normal	Abducted	Elevated
Spine	Normal	C-curve	S-curve
Rib cage	Normal	Rotated	
Pelvis	Level	Asymmetrical	
Heel alignment	Neutral	Varus	Valgus

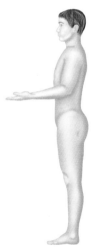

Figure 2.6: Standing view of the body, lateral view.

Head	Neutral	Forward	
Cervical spine	Normal	Hyperextension	Flat
Thoracic spine	Normal	Kyphotic	Flat
Lumbar	Normal	Lordosis	Flat
Pelvis	Neutral	Anterior tilt	Posterior tilt
Knees	Neutral	Hyperextended	Flexed
Ankle joint	Neutral	Plantar flexed	Dorsiflexed

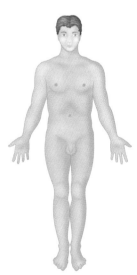

Figure 2.7: Standing view of the body, anterior view.

Arm position	Normal	Rotation (external/ internal)
Knees	Normal	Bowed/knock kneed
Feet	Normal	Pronated/supinated

Observation of Posture: Common Postural Problems.

Postural fault	Short muscles	Long muscles
Forward head position	Cervical extensors	Cervical flexors
Thoracic kyphosis	Pectoralis major/minor Triceps brachii Teres major Latissimus dorsi Anterior deltoid	Thoracic extensors Middle/lower trapezius
Anterior rotated/protracted shoulders	Upper trapezius Serratus anterior Pectoralis minor/major	Middle/lower trapezius Abdominals (external obliques)
Excessive lumbar lordosis	Lumbar erector spinae	Hip extensors
Flat back	Hip flexors	Lumbar erector spinae
Sway back	Anterior abdominals Hip extensors, upper abdominals, rectus abdominis, upper fibres of internal obliques	External obliques
Hitched hip (left)	Hip extensors, hamstrings, left lateral trunk muscles, right gluteus medius, tensor fasciae latae, piriformis, gluteus minimus	Right lateral trunk muscles, left gluteus medius, tensor fasciae latae, piriformis, gluteus minimus
Knee flexion	Hamstrings	Quadriceps, soleus
Femur (internal rotation)	*Hip medial rotators* gluteus medius/minimus, tensor fasciae latae, adductor magnus	*Hip lateral rotators* gluteus maximus, quadratus femoris, obturator internus, iliopsoas, obturator externus
Knocked knees	Iliotibial band	Adductors
Foot pronation	Peroneals	Tibialis posterior
Foot supination	Tibialis posterior	Peroneals

Movement Assessment

Following on from the postural assessment, movement assessment allows the creation of a dynamic picture of your client. It will help identify incorrect movement during the exercises as a result of muscle imbalance, altered recruitment patterns and altered muscle length and strength.

The inability to undertake the exercise will not be sufficient to illustrate movement imbalance that may be present. Results of the assessment will help you determine the selection of exercises to be undertaken in your exercise programme.

The goals of movement assessment are to:

* determine quality of movement
* identify muscle balance and endurance
* determine trunk stability
* identify muscle recruitment pattern during movement
* identify faulty movement patterns

Each test is undertaken without any hint on method or cueing/direction, and each test is repeated five times. The observer should note movement direction, quality, fluidity and control.

Walking

Purpose

To identify dynamic movement, quality of movement, movement of core areas, such as thoracic spine to lumbar spine, and lumbar spine to pelvis, balance of pelvis on weight-bearing limb, and control of trunk.

Action

• Observe the walking action from the front, back and sideways, noting movement in key points. (Key points can be noted/identified by placing a marker on the following : right/left sacroiliac joint, lumbar spine at L3 level, thoracic spine at T6 level, and on both greater tronchanter bony prominences.)

Pass criteria

Even movement with each stepping action.

Points to watch for:

Breathing faults

• abnormal/faulty/inefficient breathing pattern
• breath holding
• altered rhythm

Movement faults

• hip drop (weight-bearing/non-weight-bearing)
• altered lumbar pelvic movements (stance phase/swing through phase)
• pelvic rotation (limited/excessive)
• spinal position
• spinal rotation
• knee position
• foot movements; rolling through foot/push off

Areas of increased movement

• altered movement in lumbar pelvic area

Squat

Purpose

To assess the stability and control of the lower limbs.

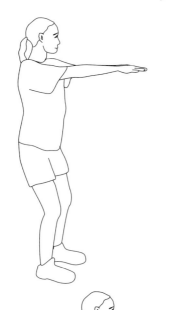

Action

- Stand with the feet shoulder-width apart and heels down.
- Keep the eyes facing forward and the shoulders square.
- Perform a squat action, with the knees aligned over the feet, and the feet facing forward. Achieve squat to 90 degrees, while the heels are kept down.

Pass criteria

Being able to squat and complete the action without restriction or discomfort.

Points to watch for:

Breathing faults

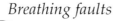

- altered pattern
- holding breath

Movement faults

- altered weight bearing
- knee position (rotation/alignment)
- limited hip flexion
- excessive lumbar spine extension
- thoracic kyphosis
- altered head position

Lunge

Purpose

To assess the dynamic stability of the lower limbs, and challenge trunk stability on combined hip extension/flexion movement.

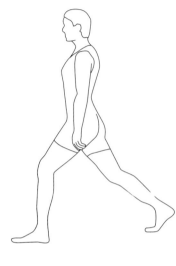

Action

- Stand with the feet shoulder-width apart and heels on the ground.
- Keep the eyes facing forward and the shoulders square.
- Step forward onto one leg, step back and alternate legs.

Pass criteria

- ability to keep the knees tracking over the toes
- keeping the front foot on the ground
- hip does not thrust forward; hip extension control
- lower back does not overarch backward
- ability to maintain balance throughout the exercise
- hip–knee control
- coordination of core areas

Points to watch for:

Breathing faults

- holding breath
- variable breathing pattern
- bracing with breath

Movement faults

- overarching of the back
- rounding the upper back forward
- pelvic rotation
- side bending of the trunk
- turning of the foot
- heel rolling
- rear leg dropping from straight leg
- returning to standing, leading movement through the body and not through the hips (pelvis)

One Leg Standing Balance

Purpose
To determine control of trunk stability while undertaking hip flexion standing.

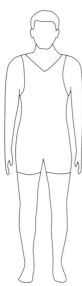

Action

- Stand with the feet hip-width apart, and fold one leg up at the hip.
- Maintain one leg standing position.

Pass criteria
Being able to hold position in one leg standing with no change in alignment of the hips (pelvis) and shoulder alignment (maintain box).

Points to watch for:

Breathing faults

- breath holding
- variable breathing pattern

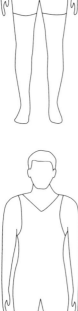

Movement faults

- trunk bracing
- altered static balance
- lack of smooth movement on hip flexion
- hip abduction (weight-bearing/non-weight-bearing sides)
- lumbo-pelvic tilting/rotation
- hip hitching/hip drop
- internal/external hip rotation
- altered ability to undertake movement in standing (Indicated by difficulty in undertaking standing activities.)

Shoulder Flexion

Purpose

To indicate shoulder stability on a stable trunk, in standing.

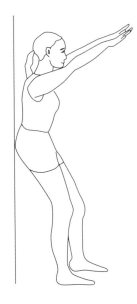

Action

- Stand with the feet shoulder-width apart and heels down.
- Keep the eyes facing forward and shoulders square.
- Place your hands together in front of your body, and lift your arms above your head.

Pass criteria

Being able to keep the trunk from moving during forward flexion of the shoulder. Being able to maintain the scapula in mid-position without scapular elevation.

Points to watch for:

Breathing faults

- breath holding
- variable breathing patterns

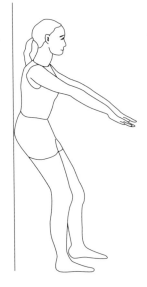

Movement faults

- trunk bracing
- lack of smooth movement
- thoraco-lumbar extension
- anterior pelvic tilting
- altered scapular positioning throughout movement

Push-up

Purpose

To determine control and strength in the shoulder girdle and trunk.

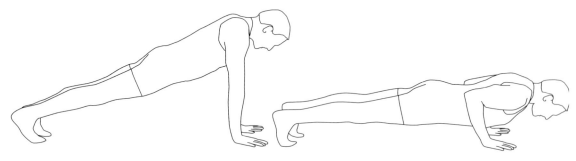

Action

- Place the wrists/elbows on the floor under the shoulders.
- Maintain a straight back, with your body weight on your toes. Bend your elbows and allow your body to move down to the floor.
- Hold the position.
- Push through your arms to straighten your elbows out.

N.B. Some people cannot complete a full push-up, and should instead place their knees on the floor.

Pass criteria

Ability to complete a push-up without substitution strategies taking place.

Points to watch for:

Breathing faults

- breath holding
- variable breathing pattern
- accessory breathing pattern

Movement faults

- trunk bracing
- altered shoulder-blade position/movement/control
- winging scapulae
- elbow hyperextension
- cervico-thoracic flexion
- upper cervical extension (head up)
- thoracic-lumbar flexion/rotation/extension
- pelvic tilting

Curl-up

Purpose

To undertake the trunk curling action in the correct sequence.

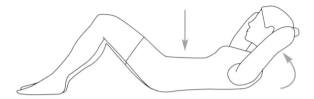

Action

- Lie flat on your back with your knees bent at 90 degrees and heels flat.
- Place your hands behind your head, with your elbows wide.
- Maintain a neutral spine.
- Curl-up and hold the position.
- Return to the floor.

Pass criteria

Being able to sequence the curl without poking your chin out or losing the pelvic neutral position.

Points to watch for:

Breathing faults

- breath holding
- variable breathing pattern from ideal (breathing out to activate the action)
- accessory breathing pattern
- bulging diaphragm

Movement faults

- lumbo-pelvic flexion/extension
- anterior pelvic tilt
- thoraco-lumbar extension
- thoracic flexion/extension
- pelvic rotation
- jarring movement
- gripping – hip flexor dominance

The Anatomy of Pilates

Four Point Challenge

Purpose

To assess the ability of the trunk to maintain a level position while being challenged.

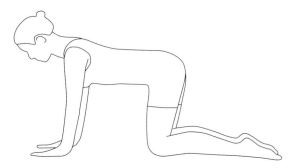

Action

- Kneel on all fours.
- Place your hands beneath your shoulders, with your knees under your hips.
- Make sure your back is in a straight line throughout the spine.
- While maintaining the spinal position in a straight line, reach out with one arm and, as a further challenge, slide the opposite leg back behind you.

Pass criteria

Being able to maintain your level back position while both the opposite leg and arm are raised.

Points to watch for:

Breathing faults

- holding breath
- variable breathing pattern

Movement faults

- inability to maintain a straight spine throughout the test
- thoracic flexion (rounding the shoulders)
- rotation in the thoracic spine
- winging of the shoulder blade
- altered scapulae position during the test; shoulder retraction on the arm lift
- forward protrusion of the head during arm lifting
- head altering position (dropping, tilting, chin poking)
- pelvic rotation

Bridge

Purpose

To challenge core stability into extension.

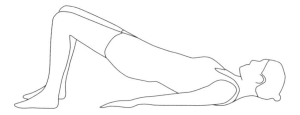

Action

- Lie on your back with your spine in neutral and knees bent at 90 degrees. Keep your feet flat on the floor.
- Lift your pelvis up off the floor, to a point where the trunk and pelvis are in a parallel line.

Pass criteria

Ability to maintain a neutral spine in the raised position. Coordination between areas.

Points to watch for:

Breathing faults

- breath holding
- variable breathing pattern
- accessory breathing pattern

Movement faults

- trunk bracing
- lumbo-pelvic rotation / tilt
- thoraco-lumbar extension–flexion–rotation
- cervico-thoracic flexion
- upper cervical extension
- altered knee extension
- cramping sensation into hamstrings

Body Alignment During Exercise

Posture
As indicated in the posture section (see page 22), there are various posture types and indicated differences in the muscles that are strong or weak. These differences result in alignment changes in the key (core) areas (neck–scapular, trunk–pelvis, etc.). There needs to be a balance between length and strength in order to complete the selected exercise(s) satisfactorily.

Leg Alignment
During the exercise, the position of the limb needs to be defined, in relation to the range and articulation of the joint being moved, by the requirements of the exercise.

Incorrect joint movement will lead to faulty joint mechanics, increased stress in the joint, and possible injury.

An example of this is excessive hip external rotation in the Leg Circles, which may result in rotation in the pelvis/lumbar spine, leading to changes in normal joint mechanics.

Head Position

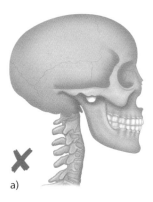 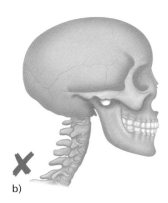 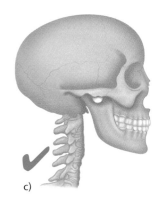

a)   b)   c)

Figure 2.8: Head and neck positioning; a) head back and down; b) head forward and down; c) head forward and up.

Finding the Position
While maintaining a loose shoulder position and soft ribs, place your head on the mat, rotate your head forward and stretch your neck, trying to flatten your neck down on the mat. Soften this position and note that the correct resting position should be between the base of the skull and the top of your head, with the forehead parallel to the ceiling. The chin should be soft and not compressing onto the throat. The sensation is one of a stretch/lengthening in your neck.

A neutral pelvis and a neutral spine are important reference points for Pilates exercises; if you are in a neutral pelvis you are in a neutral spine, with the movement of the pelvis defining the curvature in the spine.

Neutral Pelvis
Neutral pelvis is the position of your pelvis that is most natural and normal for proper body mechanics to take place. This position preserves the slight, natural curves of the spine, especially the low back, and allows your abdominals to engage properly. By gently rocking your pelvis forward and backward, you will find your neutral, a position defined by your anterior superior iliac spine (ASIS) and pubic bone being on the same plane (horizontal while lying, vertical while standing). When you find your optimal neutral position, make sure that you are also anchored to the floor at the midback. (The midback area is the core of your upper body, and when this area is anchored you are ensuring that the thoracic spine is keeping its convex curve.)

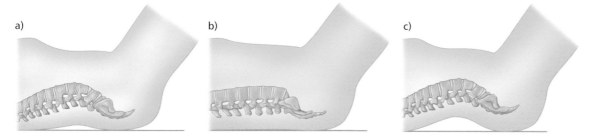

Figure 2.9: Pelvic tilt; a) neutral, where the triangle is parallel to the floor, b) posterior tilt, also know as imprint, c) anterior tilt.

Pilates originally referred to the position of the pelvis in a posterior tilt, and this continues to be of use when performing exercises where the lower limbs have no contact with the floor (open chain exercises), e.g. Single Leg Stretch. However, positioning the spine in an anterior/posterior tilt position causes increased compression on one aspect of the disc and may cause back discomfort.

Posterior Tilt = The lumbar spine flattens out and the pubic symphysis raises above the ASIS.
Anterior Tilt = The lumbar spine arches and the pubic symphysis drops below the ASIS.

Neutral Spine
A neutral spine is defined as the relative position of the anterior superior iliac spine (ASIS) and the pubic symphysis when the ASIS lies parallel in the transverse plane. Because the spine is not a straight structure, but instead has an inward curve in the cervical and lumbar areas, a neutral spine also refers to the presence of the natural curves in the spine. The neutral spine is considered a dynamic state that will move as you move through the exercise, to provide an

even load between the many joints and discs of the spine, and promote transverse abdominal strengthening. However, there are many Pilates exercises that move the spine in and out of neutral as a result of articulation and movement of the spine.

Neutral Spine/Pelvis = A natural curve results in the lumbar spine as the pubic symphysis and ASIS become level to one another.

Figure 2.10: The neutral spine position.

Rib Cage Position
The position of the rib cage and neutral spine work closely together, due to the following factors:

- the attachment of the abdominals to the ribs
- the need for good alignment of the ribs to the pelvis
- the connection to the shoulder girdle, which is a muscular connection and needed for good movement
- the importance of trunk stability

If you think of the centre of the trunk (rib cage) as the centre of the core, any restriction will lead to effects on the spine and pelvis, and alter the ability to breathe efficiently. Restricted rib movement or position, i.e. the inability of the rib cage to expand and contract with each breath, alters the movement and functional length of the spinal muscles (thoracic erector spinae group), and tightness within the latissimus dorsi.

Foot Position
When you undertake an exercise, the foot position is important to complete the posture of the lower limb and ensure the correct movement. This ensures control from the trunk and hip to the foot, which keeps the body in alignment. Two positions are used:

1. Flexed (dorsiflexed) foot. The emphasis here is to lengthen through the heels.

2. Pointed (plantar flexed) foot. This needs to be soft, not forced. A forced foot position will create unnecessary tightness and altered muscle tension.

Scapular Control
A stable shoulder girdle is essential to provide support and transfer of forces to and from the trunk, and a secure foundation for arm movement. Scapular stability is a key component of the ability to remain stable while being challenged by Pilates exercises, and is the ability to hold the shoulder girdle in neutral while using the upper limbs. Furthermore, it is the position where there is a balance between the rotator cuff muscle group and the scapular stabilizer group.

The efficiency of the scapulae to function as a core area for upper limb movement is dependent upon the activation of the stabilizer and mobilizer muscles in the correct sequence.

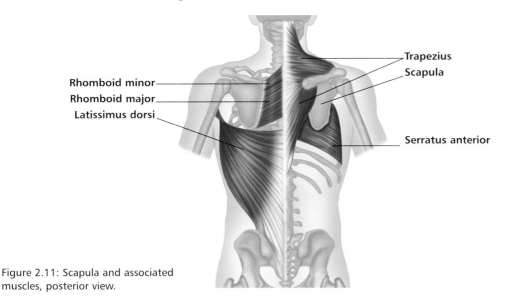

Figure 2.11: Scapula and associated muscles, posterior view.

Scapular Neutral Training
Aims

- improve positional awareness
- activate the stabilizer muscles (lower trapezius, serratus anterior)
- work the deep neck flexors

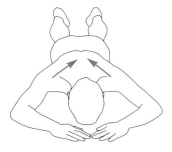

Figure 2.12: Diamond press.

Action

- Lie on your front and engage your lower abdominals.
- While breathing out, draw your shoulder blades down and back toward your waist.
- Maintain that position, and allow your head to lift, keeping the forehead parallel to the mat.
- Hold the position, then release.

Progression
Get into a four-point kneeling position, with the wrists under the shoulders. on the out-breath (engaging your lower abdominals), slide your shoulder blades down your back. At the same time, push down through your hands into the floor and pull your arms down towards your feet. Don't allow your body to move from the four-point position. Notice the engagement of the scapulae muscles and latissimus dorsi (scapular core area).

The Core/Muscle Slings

There is a functional and mechanical link between muscle groups and the core areas of movement (neck–scapular, trunk–pelvis, etc.). Due to the anatomy of key muscles, the connection of the muscles in a sling come into action to allow us to utilize our limbs and trunk in a stable, efficient and dynamic way.

This link has been labelled muscle slings. These muscle slings act as a coupling mechanism between the core areas, which allows for the transfer of force of movement between them, and are the active components in the pelvic stabilization system.

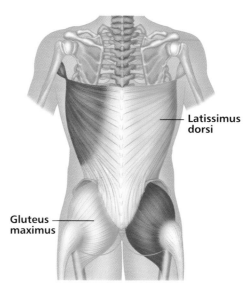

Latissimus dorsi

Gluteus maximus

Figure 2.13: The posterior oblique sling; latissimus dorsi and gluteus maximus working cooperatively.

Posterior oblique sling	Lower posterior oblique sling	Anterior oblique sling	Deep longitudinal sling	Primary sling
Gluteus maximus	Iliotibial band	Internal obliques	Myofascia of hip	Transversus abdominis
	Vastus lateralis			
Tensor fascia latae	Gluteus medius	External obliques	Biceps femoris	Multifidus
			Peroneus longus	Diaphragm
Latissimus dorsi (opposite side)	Gluteus minimus	Transversus abdominis		
	Adductors			Pelvic floor
Erector spinae		Adductors	Tibialis anterior	
Quadratus lumborum		Iliopsoas		
		Rectus abdominis		

Chapter

3

Application of the Pilates Method

Muscle Balance

Muscle Imbalance

Motor Learning

Motor Control Skills: Stabilization, Coordination

Flexibility

Strengthening

Pilates Programme

Pilates integrates the whole body, training body areas in isolation or together, through the application of movement principles and stability. Each Pilates exercise has a muscular focus (i.e. motor control, flexibility and muscle balance), or exercise objective. These areas of focus work at different progressive levels to enable the individual's ability and coordination to be built while undertaking the exercise.

Muscle Balance

Muscle balance is determined as a relationship between the tone or strength and the length of the muscles around a joint. Muscles can be broadly classified into two types: those that stabilize a joint, and those that are responsible for movement.

Stabilizers and Mobilizers
Stabilizers essentially stabilize a joint; they are made up of slow-twitch fibres for endurance, and assist with postural holding. They can be further subdivided into primary stabilizers, which have very deep attachments, lying close to the axis of rotation of the joint; and secondary stabilizers, which are powerful muscles, with an ability to absorb large amounts of force. Stabilizers work against gravity, and tend to become weak and long over time. People with poor postural alignment or an inactive lifestyle tend to have insufficient tone in these muscles.

Mobilizers are responsible for movement. They tend to be more superficial although less powerful than stabilizers, but produce a wider range of motion. They tend to cross two joints, and are made of fast-twitch fibres that produce power but lack endurance. Mobilizers assist with rapid or ballistic movement and produce high force. With time and use, they tend to tighten and shorten.

Primary stabilizers
Multifidus, transversus abdominis, internal oblique, gluteus medius, vastus medialis, serratus anterior, lower trapezius, deep neck flexors, soleus.

Secondary stabilizers
Gluteus maximus, external oblique, quadriceps, iliopsoas*, subscapularis, infraspinatus, upper trapezius*, quadratus lumborum, adductor magnus.

Mobilizers
Iliopsoas*, hamstrings, rectus femoris, tensor fasciae latae, hip adductors, piriformis, rectus abdominis, external oblique, quadratus lumborum*, erector spinae, sternocleidomastoid, upper trapezius*, levator scapulae, rhomboids, pectoralis minor, pectoralis major, scalenes, gastrocnemius.

Muscles marked with (*) can act as both stabilizers and mobilizers in different situations.

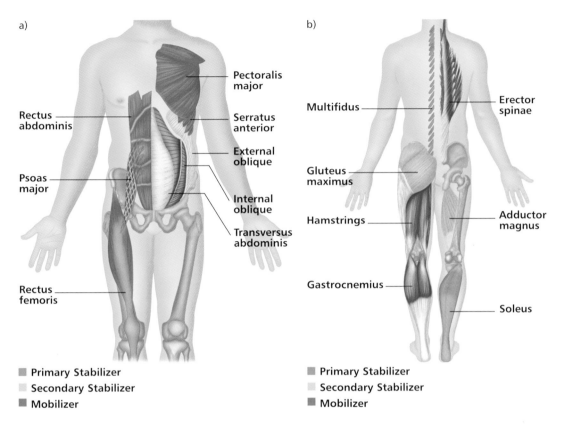

Figure 3.1: Major stabilizers and mobilizers, (a) anterior view, (b) posterior view.

So during day-to-day activity, skeletal muscles are acting as either stabilizing muscles or mobilizing muscles. As outlined above, the stabilizing muscles maintain posture or hold the body in a given position as a 'platform', so that the mobilizing muscles can cause the body to move in some way. To maintain posture, the stabilizing muscle fibres perform a minimal contraction over an extended period of time. The majority of people in modern society would benefit from exercises (such as Pilates) that specifically address their neglected deep postural muscles, as this would increase their ability to stabilize functional movements.

It is particularly important to maintain your torso as a stable platform relative to the movements carried out by your limbs. As your torso or mid-section is the 'core' of your body, its success as a stable platform is referred to as core stability. Core stability can be summarized as the successful recruitment of deep muscles that maintain the neutral (natural curvatures) position of the spine during all other movements of the body.

Furthermore, the deep stabilizing muscles collectively create what is referred to as a local unit of muscles. These muscles include the transversus abdominis, multifidis, pelvic floor, and diaphragm. The main muscles that initiate movement of the limbs while working in unison with the local muscles are

The Anatomy of Pilates

collectively referred to as the global muscles. These comprise the erector spinae, external and internal obliques, gluteals, quadratus lumborum, and rectus abdominis.

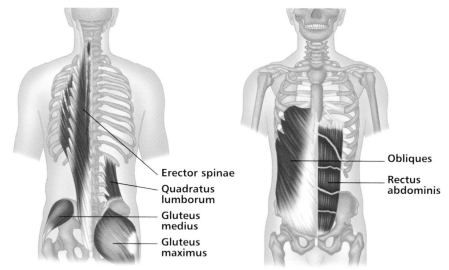

Figure 3.2: Global muscles; a) posterior view, b) anterior view.

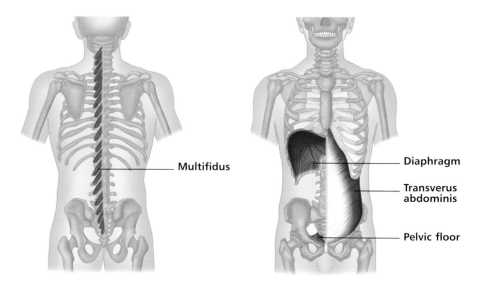

Figure 3.3: Local muscles; a) posterior view, b) anterior view.

Normal Movement Balance

The emphasis with Pilates is that the muscles should work in pairs and not in isolation. The diagram below illustrates the various roles in which muscles need to operate in order to achieve smooth movement.

As well as the activation of agonist–antagonist, they also need to work within their roles of mobilizers and stabilizers; this coordination allows for correct activation of the specific Pilates exercise.

Agonist	Synergist
Muscle that contracts to produce a specified movement.	A synergist prevents or eliminates any unwanted movement that might occur as the agonist contracts.

Antagonist	Fixator
The muscle on the opposite side of a joint to the agonist (prime mover) and which must relax to allow the prime mover to contract.	Muscle group that maintains a stable base to allow for the action of the agonist.

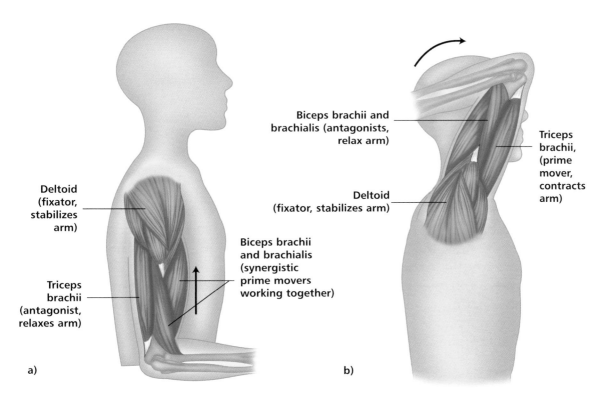

Figure 3.4: Group action of muscles: a) flexing arm at elbow, b) extending arm at elbow (showing reversed roles of prime mover and antagonist).

Muscle Imbalance

Development of Muscle Imbalance
When the muscular system is working well and in a balanced state, there will be good stability and control in the required movement; however, changes do occur. Three examples of the build-up of muscle imbalance are:

1. Over a period of time, the mobilizers can inhibit the action of the stabilizers and begin to move and attempt to stabilize on their own. This inhibition of the stabilizers and preferential recruitment of the mobilizers is central to the

build-up of muscle imbalance. In Pilates, it is noted by fixing with the external obliques, during a curl-up, in order to maintain a pelvic-neutral position.

2. Tightening of the mobilizer muscles. This will result in a limited range of motion, so altering the movement quality, and places a great stress on the joint. Tightness will result in reciprocal inhibitions (tightness in the muscle may inhibit the opposing muscle group).

3. Weakening of the stabilizer muscles. Reduction in endurance to hold a contraction can lead to lengthening of the muscle in question. Furthermore, the stabilizer muscle will reduce its ability to hold in an inner range position.

'A state of muscle imbalance exists when a muscle is weak and its antagonist is strong. The stronger of the two opponents tends to shorten, and the weaker of the two tends to elongate. Either weakness or shortness can cause faulty alignment. Weakness permits a position of deformity, but shortness creates a position of deformity.' (Kendall, 1983)

Motor Learning

The establishment of motor skill through Pilates is achieved by building the goals of stability, coordination, balance and muscle stamina (endurance), although it is now believed that some exercises may need more than 10 repetitions to build endurance. Motor learning is an adaptive response to sensory integration, using the senses of touch, vision, movement and positional sense. These form a model (an established motor development theory) comprising three phases – cognitive, associative and automatic – that integrates well with Pilates and its progressive development of exercise.

The Three Components of Adaptive Response Motor Skill Learning

Cognitive phase	Associative phase	Automatic phase
• Understand the movement. • Develop ideas on how to achieve it. • Need to focus on what movement to perform. • Need for visual input via demonstration and lots of repetition of the correct movement.	• Movement more coordinated. • More movement awareness. • Ability to cope with the challenge of new exercises. • Ability to focus on movement performance.	• Movement coordinated. • Quality in movement. • Movement automatic.
◀─────────────── **Time frame** ───────────────▶		
3 to 6 weeks	8 weeks to 4 months	Ongoing

Skills Applied to Progression of Pilates Exercises

Cognitive phase	Associative phase	Automatic phase
← —————————— Skills developed —————————— →		
Develop the breathing pattern. Establish key movement patterns – ability to identify stabilizer muscles. Ability to localize movement to core areas, together or in isolation, e.g. trunk, trunk with movement of arms/legs, etc.	Build abdominal control while being challenged. Improve movement patterns in gross form, moving from the trunk, isolated or coordinated – building use of arms/legs to challenge control of position.	Performance of complete/correct exercise with minimal attention.

Motor Control Skills: Stabilization, Coordination

Stabilization of the body during exercise is achieved through coordination and recruitment in the key or core areas. Any changes in this coordination will result in an inability to undertake the exercise. (Scapular stability is covered on page 40.)

For pelvic stability, as mentioned on page 45, the local stabilizers transversus abdominis and multifidus need to be functioning normally in partnership with the internal abdominal obliques, the diaphragm and pelvic floor. In addition to their stabilizing action, these muscles coordinate their activity during exercise to facilitate other mechanisms, such as activating other stabilizers and mobilizers to work in the correct sequencing of recruitment. Breathing patterns, pelvic floor control and trunk stability are therefore intimately connected.

Transversus abdominis connects the front and back and upper and lower halves of the body. Through these connections, it plays a role in supporting the functional movement of the upper and lower limbs as well as stabilizing the spine. It spans around the trunk, connecting into the thoraco-lumbar fascia, a thick connective tissue sheath, which helps to stabilize the trunk and pelvis.

Transversus abdominis and the thoraco-lumbar fascia provide a central corset to connect the upper and lower body, and so help to stabilize the pelvis on the spine and create a firm foundation for the leg muscles.

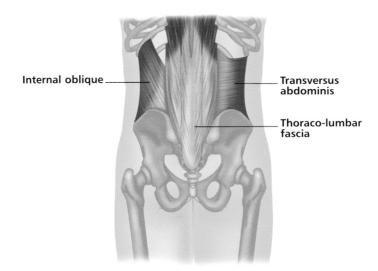

Figure 3.5: Transversus abdominis and the internal obliques inserting into the thoraco-lumbar fascia.

Stability is lost when deep stabilizing muscles have either reduced endurance to hold a contraction, or strength to hold a position against more superficial mobilizing muscles. Stability is also lost if there is a presence of muscle imbalance between large mobilizing muscle groups.

Motor Coordination
Coordination of movement is linked to the ability to undertake the exercise in a smooth, controlled manner. As motor control develops, this gradually becomes unconscious.

True motor coordination is where the principles of Pilates work together in such a way that the challenge of the movement during the exercise can be adapted. An example can be seen in the Hundred: if the challenge of straightening the leg leads to a loss of stability in the trunk–pelvis, you can decrease the load by keeping the knees bent to 90 degrees, while maintaining breathing control and upper limb movement.

Controlled intention of the movement is a gradual process, and is seen as the building up of layers of control in order to perform a natural and coordinated movement.

Flexibility

Flexibility is determined as the ability of the muscle and joint to move through their full potential range for the required activity. When the ends of the muscle attachments are moving apart, the muscle is considered to be lengthening. On the other hand, if the muscle attachments are resistant to lengthening, then the muscle would be considered to be in a shortened state.

Exercises to Lengthen Specific Muscles

Muscle	Exercise
Lower back	Double Leg Stretch, Spine Curls
Spine	Spine Curls, Roll-up, Rolling Like a Ball, Open Leg Rocker
Hamstrings	Double Leg Stretch, Scissors, Leg Circles, Open Leg Rocker
Psoas	Spine Curls, Scissors, Swimming
Quadratus lumborum	Spine Twist, Mermaid, Spine Stretch Forward
Hip abductors	Roll-up
Quadriceps	Single Leg Kick, Swimming
Gluteals	Open Leg Rocker, Seal
Piriformis	Leg Circles
Hip rotators	Leg Circles, Single Leg Kick
Tibialis anterior	Roll-up
Gastrocnemius/Soleus	Spine Stretch Forward
Rectus abdominis	Saw
Obliques	Double Leg Stretch
Latissimus dorsi	Neck Pull, Open Leg Rocker
Pectoralis major	Leg Pull Front
Neck muscles	Neck Pull

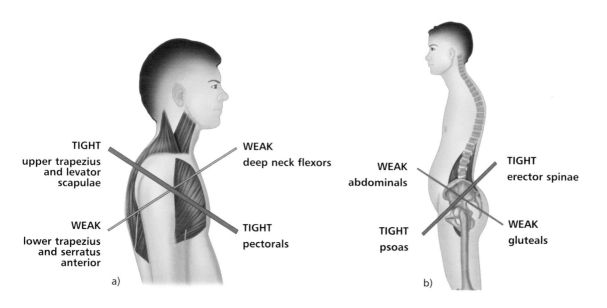

Figure 3.6: Examples of changes in muscle length/strength on posture; a) upper crossed patterns of weakness and tightness, b) lower crossed patterns of weakness and tightness.

There are a number of examples where shortened muscles can contribute to movement impairment and problems:

- muscle length is influenced by specific posture types, and differences do occur
- an inability to undertake the activity effectively
- muscle weakness
- increased risk of injury

Each exercise has an ideal muscle length that is required or fundamental to the application of a Pilates programme, and this is an indication of a good balance between mobility, strength and flexibility. Exercises that are targeted to lengthen, shorten or tighten muscles are important to establish correct movement and posture (static or dynamic).

Benefits of Flexibility

- Stretching programmes increase flexibility. Flexible muscles can improve your daily performance ability and will make functional activities and the Pilates exercises become easier and require less effort.
- Flexibility improves the range of motion of your joints. A good, functional range of motion keeps you in balance, which will help retain your mobility.
- Flexibility improves circulation, and increases blood flow to your muscles. Improved circulation can speed recovery after muscle injuries.
- Flexibility promotes better posture. Flexibility programmes help prevent your muscles from becoming tight, allowing you to maintain a good posture and reduce discomfort related to posture.
- Flexibility can relieve stress. Flexibility helps to relax tense muscles, which become associated with stressed postures.
- Flexibility may help prevent injury by preventing muscle tightness, which will alter muscle performance.

Guidelines for Flexibility Training
When a muscle has been identified as either shortened or tight, to establish good functional length, a stretching programme will need to be undertaken, before the application of a specific Pilates exercise.

Guidelines for a Stretching Programme

- Establish trunk stability (via transversus abdominis, multifidus, pelvic floor).
- Identify the muscle to be lengthened.
- Move the muscle to be lengthened through its active range to the end of the available range.
- Place gentle pressure at the end of the range. Hold for a 2-second count.
- Return the muscle to the starting position.
- Repeat the stretching movement 10 times.

Frequency	Intensity	Duration	Limitations
Minimum x2 per week. Body needs to be warm prior to stretching.	Take to end range, over pressure but not sufficient to create muscle reflex/protective tightness.	Repeat 10 times Follow with Pilates exercise that utilizes the selected muscle group.	Pain on active movement to the tension point. Joint/muscle injury, undiagnosed.

Key Points

Don't bounce, because bouncing stimulates the tension–stretch reflex mechanisms which, once activated, protect the muscle from damage and any increase in range of motion.

Focus on pain-free stretching/lengthening. Expect to feel tension at the end of the active phase during the stretch movement. If it hurts, you have gone too far. You only need to take the movement to the first tight point and not into the tight area.

Relax and breathe freely. Don't hold your breath while you stretch.

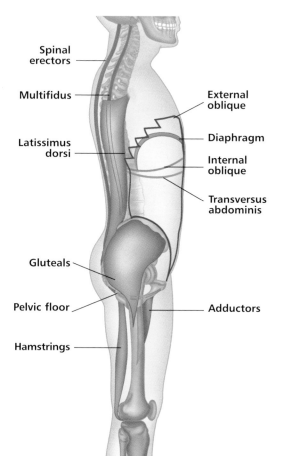

Spinal erectors

Multifidus

Latissimus dorsi

External oblique

Diaphragm

Internal oblique

Transversus abdominis

Gluteals

Pelvic floor

Adductors

Hamstrings

Strengthening

Trunk muscle strengthening is also referred to in the fitness industry as core strength/stability. As previously indicated see page 12), core stability is illustrated in Pilates by the term 'powerhouse'.

Pilates programmes work on a sequence of movements that build muscular strength. When undertaking Pilates exercises, it is necessary to undertake a flowing sequence of muscle/movement components in order to achieve the ideal exercise technique.

You need to be able to isolate and contract the core stabilizer muscles, and then train them to work. When you are able to isolate the deep stabilizer muscles and maintain control in this group, the mobilizer muscles can then be utilized in the movement pattern required for the

Figure 3.7: Lateral view of the core stability muscles.

exercise concerned. (These points need to be understood before undertaking any of the classical exercises described later in Chapter 4.)

Pilates exercises try to develop from stabilizer–core muscles, rather than being a pure strengthening programme.

The programme is progressive due to the sequenced activation of muscle groups (development works initially with the stabilizer and then the mobilizer muscle groups, both at a local level and a global level), and the neural pathway connections made (by performing the exercise correctly each time and in the right pattern).

The challenge from Pilates comes from:

- Working from a stable neutral spine that is connected to the rib position (trunk position) and correct shoulder alignment.
- Being able to maintain this correct alignment of the core areas while undertaking exercise/movement.
- Progressively increasing the involvement of the limbs.
- Increasing the involvement and length of the limbs with the exercise.
- Working on the ability to control the correct movement in an efficient manner. Movement at speed and/or as haphazard movement is not relevant when undertaking Pilates – performing the exercise correctly is the goal.
- Increasing the complexity of the spatial pattern of the motion of the limbs, e.g. linear pattern of the leg in the Single Leg Stretch, and the rotational pattern in Leg Circles.
- Altering the rhythm and pace of the exercise.
- Altering the complexity of the exercise programme sequence, within ability, so that the programme undertaken can involve the whole classical mat programme rather than parts, i.e. Series of Five: (Single Leg Stretch, Double Leg Stretch, Single Straight Leg Stretch, Double Straight Leg Stretch, Criss-cross).
- Direction of movement.

The correct sequence of the exercise allows the right muscles to operate on demand as required.

Muscle Groups

As previously indicated, muscles work either together or in opposition to achieve movement through the joint. Before and during Pilates exercises, it is necessary to train antagonist–agonist pairings of muscles to work in an integrated and coordinated way in order to achieve smooth, fluid movement, and reduce the potential for injury.

Altered Performance
Altered performance is due to a number of reasons that can be seen in isolation or combination, which can result in a failure to perform the exercise.

Reasons for Inability to Perform the Exercise

| Musculo-skeletal | | Respiratory | Neural |
Articular components	Muscle components		Motor control and integration
Joint stiffness	Muscle inhibition	Altered breathing pattern due to incorrect muscle activity (overuse of oblique muscle group)	Muscle inhibition
Inflammation of joint	Muscle weakness/ atrophy		Alteration in muscle tone
Joint instability	Reduced muscle endurance		Poor muscle sequencing/ patterning
		Inefficiency	
	Muscle or neural tissue contraction/ tightness (muscle stiffness)	Hyperventilation	Unconscious and conscious control imbalance
	Muscle imbalance		Decreased mental conditioning
			Reduced perceptual skills

Factors That Contribute to Muscle Weakness and Alter Performance

1. Muscle atrophy
This type of weakness is illustrated by the inability of the muscle to hold the position required, which may be due to lack of use. Note the muscle effort in the push-up exercise in the scapular area, when maintaining this position.

Improvement in this weakness is achieved by training the specific muscles required to undertake the exercise.

2. Muscle strain
A strain to a muscle is indicated by the presence of pain when the muscle is contracted. This results from the muscle fibres tearing due to the inability to cope with the demands placed upon them. There are three grades of muscle strain.

Grade one strains are indicated by a small number of torn fibres, with localized pain and no loss of strength.

Grade two strains are indicated by a significant number of torn fibres, with pain when contracting the muscle, reduced strength, and limited movement (due to pain).

Grade three strains are indicated by a complete tear of the muscle (seen mostly at the musculo-tendinous junction).

There is no place in a Pilates programme for the occurrence of muscle strain. For this to occur would indicate that you are working at an excessive level in relation to your ability and load capability.

3. Muscle soreness
This is seen to accompany muscle strain due to a chemical present in the muscle tissue. One type is delayed onset muscle soreness, or DOMS. This develops as a dull ache 24–48 hours after exercise and may last for three days. It appears to be worse with eccentric exercise (involving muscle contraction while the muscle is lengthening).

The true cause is unknown, but factors that seem to help are a correct warm-down after exercise, undertaking active, non-weight-bearing exercise, and applying warmth into the muscle, e.g. by warm baths.

4. Muscle cramp
This is an involuntary condition resulting in suddenly painful muscles and an inability to undertake the muscle contraction. There are a number of theories on why it occurs, such as dehydration, low sodium levels and excessively tight muscles.

There are no guaranteed strategies, but prevention may be achieved by:

- regular specific muscle stretching, maintaining normal muscle tissue length
- correction of muscle balance and posture
- adequate conditioning for the activity by use of exercise recovery periods
- eccentric muscle strengthening into training programme, achieved in a comprehensive Pilates programme

5. Muscle weakness due to overstretching
If a muscle is maintained in a lengthened position for a prolonged period of time, that muscle becomes weak, denoted by poorly sustained postures and poor exercise technique. This overstretching can be reversed if you undertake strengthening of the muscle with alternate exercises that utilize similar muscle groups, and correct the relevant factors that have lead to the overstretching, e.g. slumping while sitting.

6. Muscle stiffness
This is determined as the ratio of the force change to length change in the muscle during movement. The two components that make up stiffness are:

1. Intrinsic muscle stiffness: the physical make-up of the muscle.

2. Reflex-mediated stiffness: the sensory and motor control system of the muscle spindle, which is sensitive to changes in length and force at a muscle fibre level.

Changes to these two components will affect your ability to move well, in a coordinated, flowing manner.

Pilates Programme

Sequence of Pilates Movement
When undertaking a Pilates exercise, it is necessary to undertake a flowing sequence of muscle–movement components in order to achieve the ideal exercise technique. You need to be able to isolate and contract the core stabilizer muscles, and train them to work.

Each exercise can be broken down into movement components in order to achieve the specific goal of the exercise, and should be in repetitions as described in the table on page 60, depending on the complexity of the exercise. For practising a static hold of the neutral position, you should be able to repeat 10 times, with a 10-second hold each time.

The ability to engage the core and its control is a dynamic process, as is the ability to maintain spinal alignment with the same quality of control of the pelvis. This dynamic process is also needed to control the pelvis to establish a stable base from which to work. It is not just about abdominal strength, but a coordinated, controlled contraction of the abdominals that responds to the demands placed upon it. The more superficial muscles (or mobilizer muscle groups) need to work on the same stable base, so the deep stabilizer muscles (transversus abdominis, gluteus minimus/medius, and scapular stabilizers) need to have the correct activation and endurance ability to meet the challenges of the Pilates exercises.

Further contraction of the core (stabilizing) abdominals in the preparation phase for all the exercises may be required if the limbs are to create the force.

When you are able to isolate the deep stabilizer muscles and maintain control in this group, the mobilizer muscles can then be utilized in the movement pattern required for the exercise undertaken.

The Anatomy of Pilates

Summary of a Pilates Exercise Used in a Stability Programme for the Trunk

Stage one	Stage two	Stage three
Isolate and train deep stabilizer muscles.	Maintain deep stabilizers, isolate muscles in the outer muscle group of the muscle sling used in that exercise. Gradually increase the load on the deep stabilizer muscles (move limbs).	Make the exercise more complex while maintaining the deep stabilizer muscles (core). Build the speed.
Transversus abdominis. Multifidus. Pelvic floor.	Muscle sling: Posterior/anterior oblique. Deep longitudinal. Primary.	Most mobilizing muscles.

(Adapted from: Richardson, C. et al., 1998).

These points need to be considered before undertaking any of the classical exercises set out in Chapter 4.

Components of Each Exercise

	Preparing to move	Initiating movement	Peak of movement effort	Return phase
Focus of muscle activity	Isometric	Eccentric	Concentric	Eccentric
Breathing pattern Each exercise may have a specific breathing pattern, due to complexity of the exercise	Breathe in	Breathe out	Hold/Breathe in	Breathe out
Muscle group activation	Deep stabilizers	Mobilizers	Global stabilizers	Mobilizers
Stabilization	Neutral position	Increasing	Peak effort	Reducing to base level
Load	Low	Increase	Maximum for exercise	Reducing
Coordination	Low	Medium	High	Medium

Exercise Selection

When selecting exercises to undertake, there are a number of considerations to be made.

1. Start by applying the Pilates principles to create a stable start position. (This may be the neutral spine position on the mat.) Undertake quality contraction of the core stabilizer muscles, and maintain movement awareness and the correct alignment. Enhance your breathing pattern.

2. Know the goal of each exercise.

3. During the main phase of the exercise, maintain muscle balance, a flowing, quality movement, and stability before mobility.

Pilates exercises follow a sequence of development, which is indicated in the order of the classical programme, but once a stable base has been established, it may be of use to work in specific directions or patterns to help the overall movement development. Here are some suggestions of exercises divided into directions.

Movement Patterns and Exercise Selection

Movement patterns	Exercise selection
Spinal flexion	Spine Curls Roll-up Spine Stretch Forward Hundred, Series of Five
Spinal extension	Swan Dive Double Leg Kick
Spinal rotation/side flexion	Mermaid, Saw, Spine Twist Single Leg Series
Pelvis–hip joint, mobilization and muscle strengthening	Spine Curls, Leg Circles Spine Stretch Forward, Torpedo
Upper body strengthening and stabilization	Double Leg Stretch, Hundred Leg Pull Front

The Anatomy of Pilates

Selection of Pilates Exercises Based on Level of Ability

Exercise	Level	Repetitions
Hundred	B	100 beats
Roll-up	B	3 reps
Rollover	A	5 each way
Single Leg Circles	B	5 each way
Rolling Like a Ball	B	6 reps
Single Leg Stretch	B	5 sets
Double Leg Stretch	B	6 reps
Single Straight Leg Stretch/Scissors	I	5 sets
Double Straight Leg Stretch	I	5 reps
Criss-cross	I	5 sets
Spine Stretch Forward	B	3 reps
Open Leg Rocker	I	6 reps
Corkscrew	A	3 sets
Saw	I	3 sets
Swan Dive	A	6 reps
Single Leg Kick	I	6 sets
Double Leg Kick	A	5sets
Neck Pull	I	3 reps
Scissors	A	3 sets
Bicycle	A	5 sets each way
Shoulder Bridge	A	3 sets
Spine Twist	I	3 sets
Jack Knife	A	3 reps
Side Kick Lift	B	3sets
Teaser	I	3 reps
Hip Circles	A	3R, 3L
Swimming	I	20 strokes
Leg Pull Front	A	3 sets
Leg Pull Back	A	3 sets
Side Kick Kneeling	A	4R, 4L
Spine Twist	A	3R, 3L
Boomerang	A	6 reps
Seal	B	6 reps
Control and Balance	A	6 sets
Push-up	A	3 reps

B = Beginner; I = Intermediate; A = Advanced.

Chapter

4

Classical Pilates Exercises

The hundred

Roll-up

Rollover

Single leg circles

Rolling like a ball

Single leg stretch

Double leg stretch

Single straight leg
   stretch

Double straight leg
   stretch

Criss-cross

Spine stretch forward

Open leg rocker

Double leg circles
   (cork screw)

Saw

Swan dive

Single leg kick

Double leg kick

Neck pull

Scissors

Bicycle

Shoulder bridge

Spine twist

Jack knife

Side kick lift

Side-lying leg circles

Torpedo

Teaser

Hip circles

Swimming

Leg pull front

Leg pull back

Side kick kneeling

The twist

Boomerang

Seal

Rocking

Control and balance

Push-up

Mermaid

Spine curls

Footnote

*Under the 'muscle focus' heading, the muscles have been mainly listed within their respective grouping,
such as hamstrings, or by movement, such as hip flexors. This is because an exercise may use one or more
than one muscle within each.*

THE HUNDRED

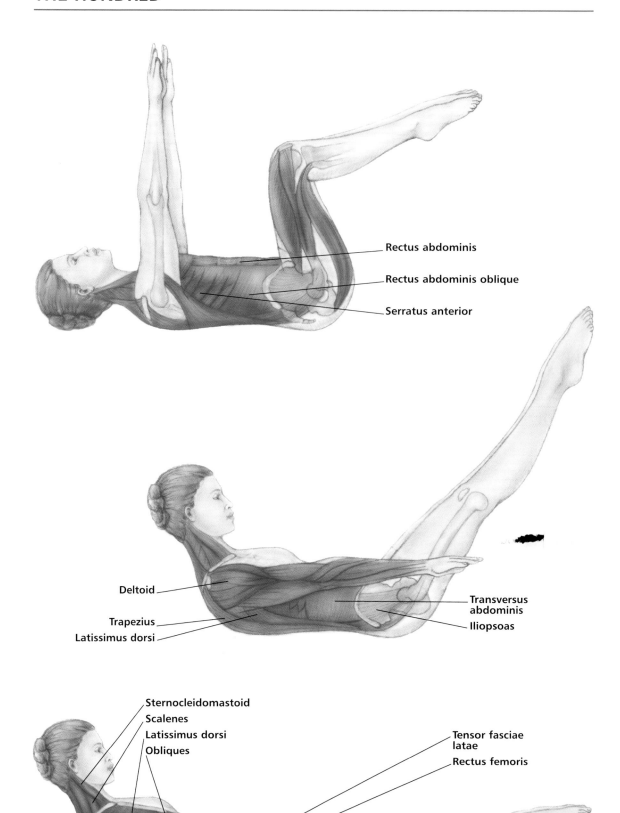

Rectus abdominis

Rectus abdominis oblique

Serratus anterior

Deltoid

Trapezius

Latissimus dorsi

Transversus abdominis

Iliopsoas

Sternocleidomastoid

Scalenes

Latissimus dorsi

Obliques

Tensor fasciae latae

Rectus femoris

Objectives of exercise

Enhance strength in the abdominal muscle group. Improve breathing control and the use of thoracic breathing pattern. Stimulate circulation and as a warm-up exercise.

Exercise description

- Lie on your back with knees bent at 90 degrees, arms reaching up to the ceiling, and palms down.
- Roll up from the top of your head, reaching the hand down behind your feet, and palms down.
- Straighten your legs and connect your heels together, pointing to a fixed point. Maintain this point with the feet turned out. As you progress your abdominal strength, you can lower the legs.
- Pump your arms on a count of five, coordinating your breathing with the arm pump action, and the hands reaching long, off the floor.

Cues to exercise

Imagine a ball under your chin, held lightly, to maintain the correct head position. Work on your breathing through the ribs (lateral breathing).

Breathing pattern

Exhale: five arm pumps. *Inhale*: five arm pumps.

Checkpoints

- Maintain your spine in the neutral position.
- Work at a level to complement your abdominal strength.
- Completely empty your lungs with each exhalation.
- Maintain the connection of the shoulders to the trunk throughout.

Pitfalls

- Losing control in the correct head position.
- Allowing your shoulders to roll forward.
- Trunk movement with arm pumps; you need to maintain a static trunk.
- Maintain low eye line (watch your abdominals do not bulge).

Muscle focus

Abdominal muscle group. Deep neck flexors. Hip flexors. Serratus anterior.

ROLL-UP

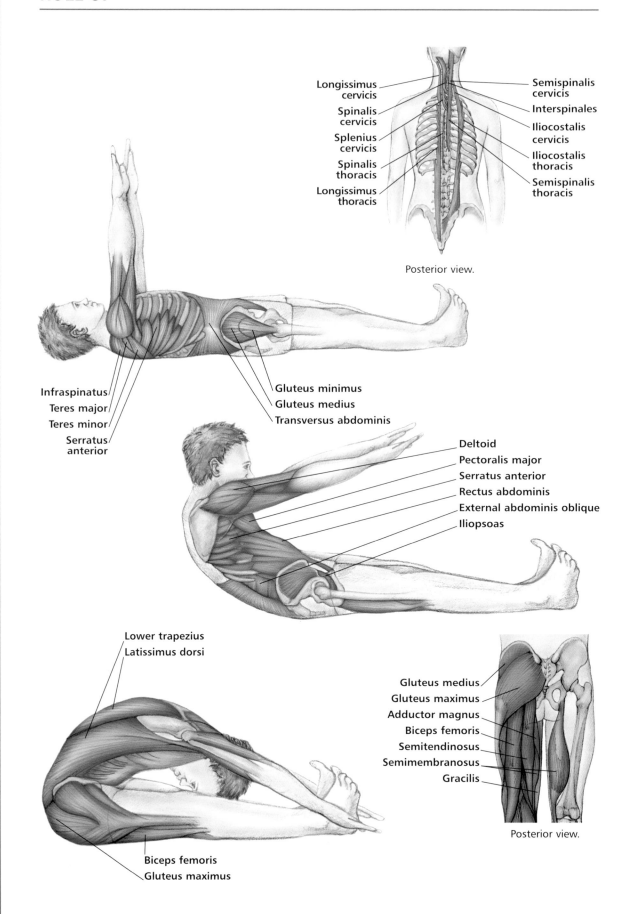

Longissimus cervicis

Spinalis cervicis

Splenius cervicis

Spinalis thoracis

Longissimus thoracis

Semispinalis cervicis

Interspinales

Iliocostalis cervicis

Iliocostalis thoracis

Semispinalis thoracis

Posterior view.

Infraspinatus

Teres major

Teres minor

Serratus anterior

Gluteus minimus

Gluteus medius

Transversus abdominis

Deltoid

Pectoralis major

Serratus anterior

Rectus abdominis

External abdominis oblique

Iliopsoas

Lower trapezius

Latissimus dorsi

Gluteus medius

Gluteus maximus

Adductor magnus

Biceps femoris

Semitendinosus

Semimembranosus

Gracilis

Posterior view.

Biceps femoris

Gluteus maximus

Objectives of exercise

Strengthen the abdominals. Restore normal timing in the lumbar spine. Lengthen the hamstrings. Develop spinal mobility and stability. Stretch the muscles of the back.

Exercise description

- Lie on your back with your arms above your head.
- Relax your ribs on the floor, elbows straight, legs extended and the heels pressed into the ground.
- Engage the lower stomach muscles to create a slight tension in your hips' abductors.
- Stretch your arms out above your head and begin to roll up.
- Continue to roll up until your hands reach a point above your feet.
- Reverse the movement, keeping your stomach muscles engaged until your shoulders blades reach the floor and your arms return to the same point above your head. Lower your head to complete the movement.
- Work on your breathing through the ribs (lateral breathing).

Cues to exercise

Push through the heels. Keep looking down throughout the exercise. Keep the abdominals engaged throughout. Move through each vertebra one by one. Maintain your neck in a long and relaxed position to minimize the tension in your upper body. Work on peeling your spine off the mat.

Breathing pattern

Breathe in to prepare. Breathe out on the roll up. Breathe in when you are in the stretched position. Breathe out when you return to the start position.

Checkpoints

- On the roll down, relax the front aspect of your hips (don't grip), and keep the front of the hips soft.
- Keep the chest soft.
- Open the shoulders on the roll down.
- On the return movement, initial the movement by softening the breastbone.
- Do not hold your breath.
- Maintain softness in the arms.
- Maintain a smooth roll throughout.

Pitfalls

- Losing control of your abdominals.
- Poking your chin upwards.
- Flopping back on the floor on the return movement.
- Allowing your feet or legs to lift off the floor as you roll up.

Muscle focus

Back extensors. Latissimus dorsi. Gluteals. Hamstrings. Abdominals. Obliques. Iliopsoas.

ROLLOVER

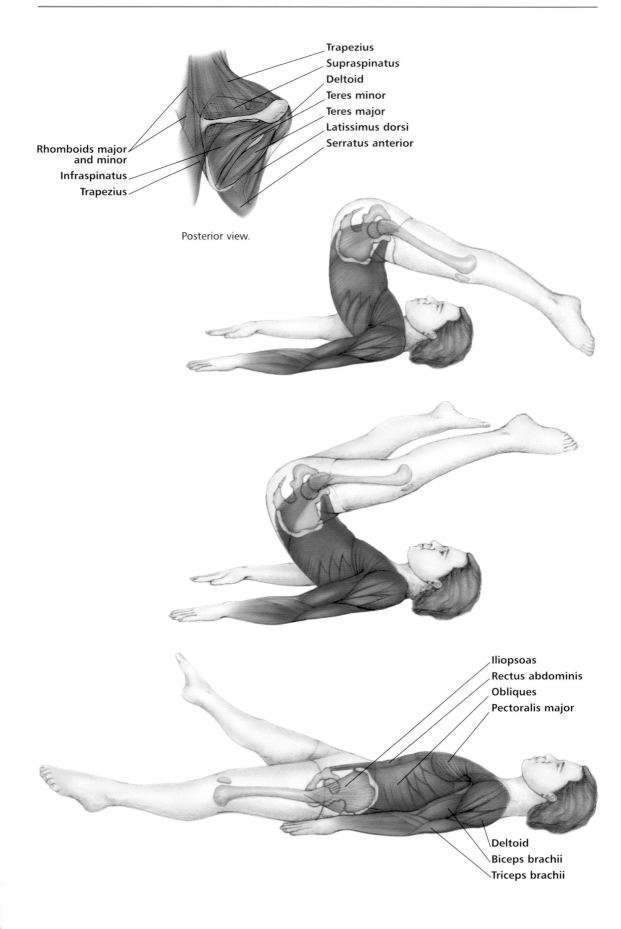

Trapezius
Supraspinatus
Deltoid
Teres minor
Teres major
Latissimus dorsi
Serratus anterior

Rhomboids major and minor
Infraspinatus
Trapezius

Posterior view.

Iliopsoas
Rectus abdominis
Obliques
Pectoralis major

Deltoid
Biceps brachii
Triceps brachii

Objectives of exercise

Control and challenge your spinal flexibility. Deep control/contraction of the abdominals and back muscles. Lengthen the spine. Allow articulation of the spine. Stretch to lower back and hamstrings.

Exercise description

- Lie flat on the floor with your arms at your side and slowly raise your legs off the mat, continuing to take the straight leg over your head to touch the floor with your toes. Maintain the pressure into the floor with your arms.
- Spread your legs hip-width apart, and then slowly roll your spine back down onto the floor; maintain the straight leg throughout the return. Bring them together as your feet approach the mat.
- In a controlled manner, return the legs together to the starting position.

Cues to exercise

Engage your lower stomach muscles before you start lowering your legs.

Breathing pattern

Breathe out when you raise the legs up. Breathe in when turning the toes to the floor. Breathe out when returning the legs to the start position.

Checkpoints

- Maintain movement at a steady pace in both directions.
- Work the abdominals throughout the exercise.
- Maintain an open chest, with the arms reaching down past your hips.
- Keep your head still.
- Don't let your knees turn inward during the exercise.
- Maintain a long neck with the base of the skull on the mat.

Pitfalls

- Using momentum to achieve roll over.
- Losing the 90-degree angle maintained in the hips during the roll over.
- Not maintaining the thighs close to the chest in the roll back phase.
- Rolling too far onto your neck.

Muscle focus

Iliopsoas. Rectus abdominis. Obliques. Shoulder flexors. Shoulder extensors.

SINGLE LEG CIRCLES

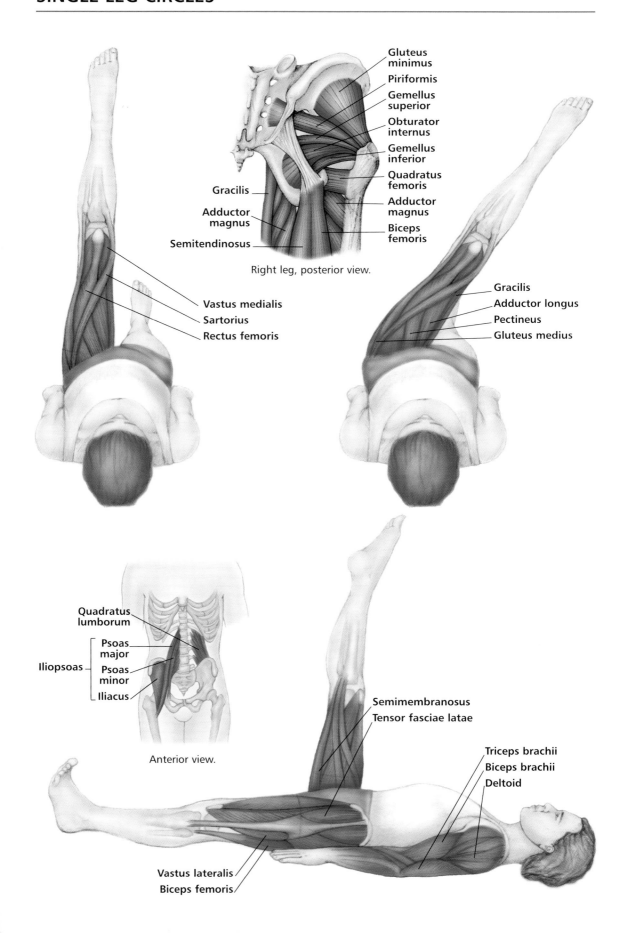

Gluteus minimus
Piriformis
Gemellus superior
Obturator internus
Gemellus inferior
Quadratus femoris
Adductor magnus
Biceps femoris
Gracilis
Adductor magnus
Semitendinosus

Right leg, posterior view.

Vastus medialis
Sartorius
Rectus femoris

Gracilis
Adductor longus
Pectineus
Gluteus medius

Quadratus lumborum
Iliopsoas
Psoas major
Psoas minor
Iliacus

Anterior view.

Semimembranosus
Tensor fasciae latae

Triceps brachii
Biceps brachii
Deltoid

Vastus lateralis
Biceps femoris

Objectives of exercise

Improve stability through the trunk. Work abdominals, especially obliques, to maintain trunk stability during the circles. Achieve stability of the neutral pelvis. Improve your ability to move, in a controlled manner, the leg separately from the pelvis. Develop control of the hip flexors.

Exercise description

- Lie on your back with your arms at your side.
- Raise one leg as high as you can, keeping your back on the mat.
- Keep both legs straight.
- Make a circle with your leg, moving it across your body, down toward the mat, out and up.
- Do three circles, and then change direction.

Cues to exercise

Start with small circles and increase the size slowly. Relax the hip flexors so that the leg can move freely.

Breathing pattern

Breathe out for the first half of the circle. Breathe in while you swing your leg up to the starting position.

Checkpoints

- Maintain a straight leg. (If necessary, the exercise can be undertaken with a bent knee, raised.)
- Maintain the lower back on the mat. (Movement is in the hip and not the lumbar spine.)
- Maintain the pelvis in the neutral position throughout the exercise.
- Don't take any strain into the neck – maintain a long neck.
- Keep the palms down to prevent the body from rocking from side to side.
- Control the circles of your leg to keep the movement in the hip and not the back.

Pitfalls

- Body movement.
- Strain in the neck.
- Loss of control of a neutral pelvis.

Muscle focus

Hip flexors. Hamstrings. Adductors. Abductors. Hip rotators. Arm extensors.

ROLLING LIKE A BALL

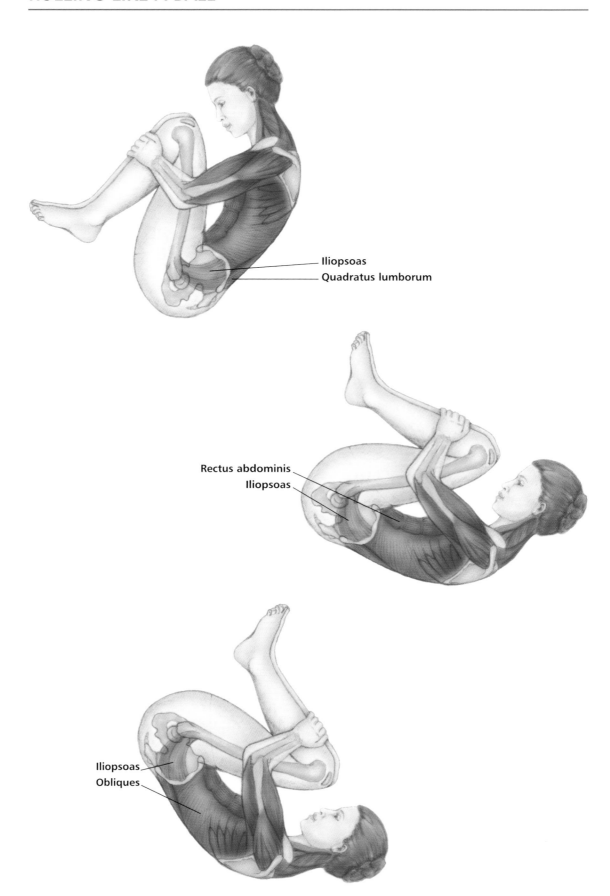

Iliopsoas
Quadratus lumborum

Rectus abdominis
Iliopsoas

Iliopsoas
Obliques

Objectives of exercise

Reduce tension in the spine. Gain and establish control of the balance point. Establish control of the momentum of the movement. Challenge the ability to maintain abdominal contraction throughout the exercise.

Exercise description

- Sit on the edge of your mat, and establish your balance point.
- Bend your knees until your feet touch your buttocks. Place your hands around the front of your knees.
- Tucking your chin into your chest, contract your abdominals.
- Allow your body to roll backward bringing your feet with you.
- Keep your elbows wide.
- As you roll back, maintain the distance between your chest and your thighs. Make sure that you keep your heels close to your buttocks throughout the exercise.
- Allow your body to roll back to the starting position using your gluteals to help create momentum.

Cues to exercise

Think massage of your back as you roll back. Allow your momentum to help you roll backward. Pinch your buttocks together as you scoop to roll: this helps to control the balance point.

Breathing pattern

Breathe in to prepare. Breathe out as you begin the movement. Breathe in as you return.

Checkpoints

- Open your knees slightly initially to help the control of the movement.
- Don't let your back thump against the floor on the roll back; use your abdominals to articulate the spine, pressing your spine into the mat to make a smooth movement.
- Don't hunch the shoulders up; keep them connected through the trunk.
- Maintain the abdominals throughout the movement.
- Keep chin to chest.

Pitfalls

- Allowing your abdominals to relax, which you need to maintain throughout the exercise.
- Rolling too far back and placing a stress on your neck.
- Thumping against the floor. Slow down the movement, and work on scooping your abdominals.

Muscle focus

Iliopsoas. Rectus abdominis. Obliques.

SINGLE LEG STRETCH

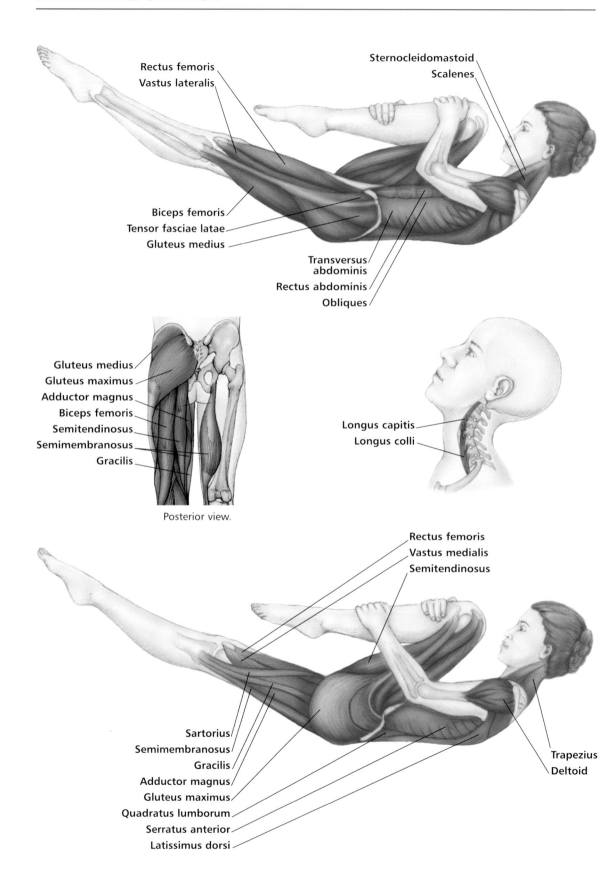

Rectus femoris
Vastus lateralis
Sternocleidomastoid
Scalenes
Biceps femoris
Tensor fasciae latae
Gluteus medius
Transversus abdominis
Rectus abdominis
Obliques

Gluteus medius
Gluteus maximus
Adductor magnus
Biceps femoris
Semitendinosus
Semimembranosus
Gracilis

Posterior view.

Longus capitis
Longus colli

Rectus femoris
Vastus medialis
Semitendinosus

Sartorius
Semimembranosus
Gracilis
Adductor magnus
Gluteus maximus
Quadratus lumborum
Serratus anterior
Latissimus dorsi

Trapezius
Deltoid

Objectives of exercise

Achieve stability of movement. Coordinate movement. Gain control of the deep abdominal muscles.

Exercise description

- Lie on your back with your knees folded onto your chest. Your knees should be at 90 degrees with your toes together and slightly pointed.
- Place your hands on the outside of your calves. Your head should be resting on the floor.
- Engage your lower abdominals and slowly curl up your head. Place your right hand on the outside of your right ankle. Place your left hand on the inside of your right knee.
- Stretch your left leg away from your body, keeping it straight. Keep the foot soft. As you stretch your left leg away, fold your right knee closer to your chest. Alternate arms–leg position.

Cues to exercise

Ensure that the straight leg only goes as low as necessary to maintain control through the trunk. (Take care not to strain the lower back.) Maintain the curl-up position throughout the exercise. Keep the elbows wide and take care not to slump into the exercise.

Breathing pattern

Breathe in to prepare on the leg change over phase. Breathe out on the outward movement.

Checkpoints

- If the neck starts to strain, lower the head toward the mat.

Pitfalls

- Not maintaining your deep abdominal control throughout the movement.
- Losing your neutral pelvis position.
- Developing tension in your neck and shoulder.
- Keep the length even on both sides of the trunk. (Don't make the mistake of leaning toward one side so that the trunk is shifting.)

Muscle focus

Hamstrings. Gluteals. Latissimus dorsi. Obliques. Quadratus lumborum. Abdominals. Deep neck flexors. Scapular stabilizers. Hip flexors. Hip extensors (gluteus maximus).

DOUBLE LEG STRETCH

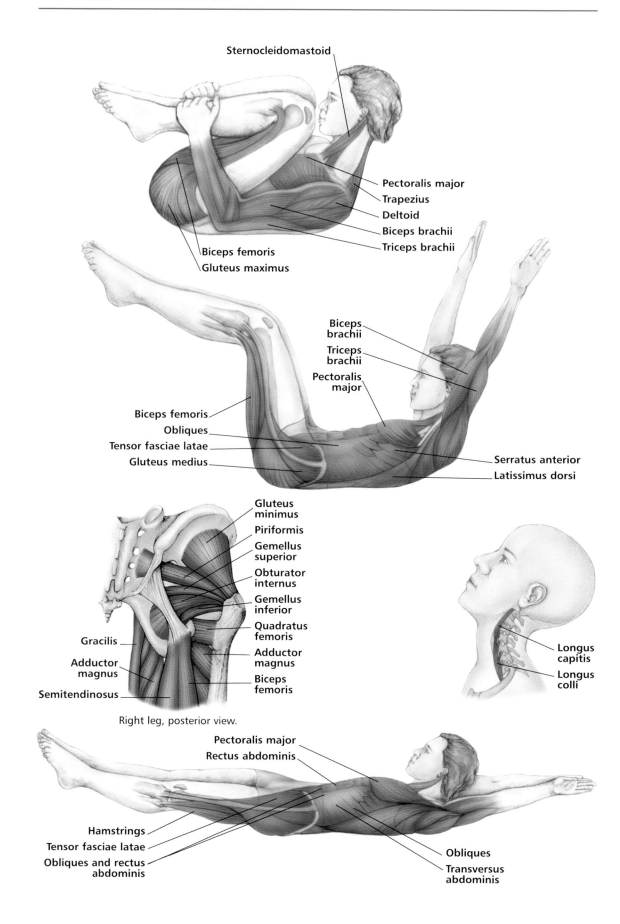

Sternocleidomastoid

Pectoralis major
Trapezius
Deltoid
Biceps brachii
Triceps brachii

Biceps femoris
Gluteus maximus

Biceps
brachii
Triceps
brachii
Pectoralis
major

Biceps femoris
Obliques
Tensor fasciae latae
Gluteus medius

Serratus anterior
Latissimus dorsi

Gluteus
minimus
Piriformis
Gemellus
superior
Obturator
internus
Gemellus
inferior
Quadratus
femoris
Adductor
magnus
Biceps
femoris

Gracilis
Adductor
magnus
Semitendinosus

Right leg, posterior view.

Longus
capitis
Longus
colli

Pectoralis major
Rectus abdominis

Hamstrings
Tensor fasciae latae
Obliques and rectus
abdominis

Obliques
Transversus
abdominis

Objectives of exercise

Strengthen the abdominals while moving the centre of gravity. Strengthen the deep neck flexors. Coordinate your breathing throughout the sequence. Enhance trunk stability. Build coordination and flowing movement.

Exercise description

- Lie on your back with your knees on your chest, hold your knees with your hands, with the knees hip-width apart, and toes together.
- Slowly curl your trunk to lengthen, and lift the back of your neck off the mat.
- Straighten your legs so that they are turned away from the hips, and heels together.
- Flex your feet and feel your legs lengthen through your heels.
- At the same time as lengthening your legs, take your arms up into a wide sweep until they are level with your ears.
- Circle your arms back round to your thighs.
- Lower your head to the starting position and bend your knees.
- Repeat the sequence.

Cue to exercise

Maintain a stable base throughout the exercise.

Breathing pattern

Breathe in to prepare. Breathe out as you stretch your arms and legs away from the starting position. Breathe in as you return to the starting position.

Checkpoints

- Keep the spine in neutral throughout the exercise.
- Don't allow your back to arch.
- Keep your abdominals pulled in throughout the exercise. Initially keep your legs high as your abdominal strength develops, maintaining control throughout the exercise.
- Keep your inner thighs connected when you lengthen the legs away.
- Keep your shoulders connected throughout the exercise.
- Maintain an open chest. (Don't fold into the chest as you raise your head.)

Pitfalls

- Allowing your abdominals to lose control during the exercise.
- Poking your chin out during the exercise.
- Taking your arms beyond your ears. (This will cause your rib cage to rise and increase the loss of control over your trunk.)

Muscle focus

Latissimus dorsi. Pectorals. Abdominals. Obliques. Deep neck flexors. Adductors. Psoas. Lower trapezius. Gluteals. Hamstrings. External hip rotators. Arm rotators.

SINGLE STRAIGHT LEG STRETCH

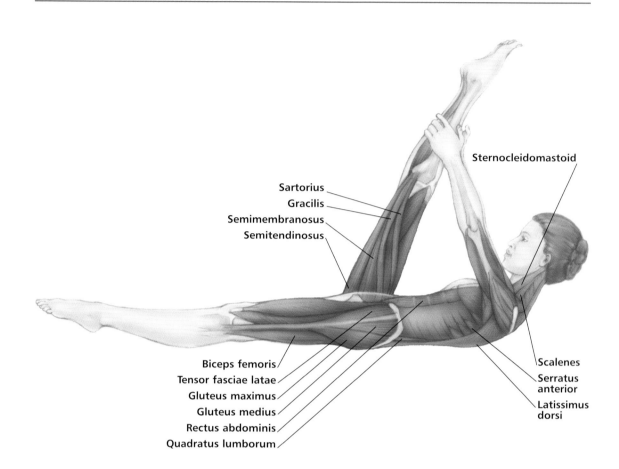

Sartorius
Gracilis
Semimembranosus
Semitendinosus

Sternocleidomastoid

Scalenes
Serratus anterior
Latissimus dorsi

Biceps femoris
Tensor fasciae latae
Gluteus maximus
Gluteus medius
Rectus abdominis
Quadratus lumborum

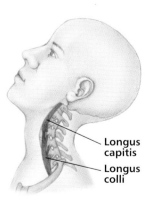

Longus capitis
Longus colli

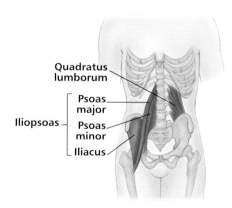

Quadratus lumborum
Psoas major
Iliopsoas
Psoas minor
Iliacus

Anterior view.

Objectives of exercise

Lengthen the back of the thigh. Improve control and strength through the legs. Increase strength in the abdominals. Improve the ability to move the leg separately from the trunk.

Exercise description

- Curl up from the mat.
- Stretch one leg out and extend the opposite leg so that it is just off the floor. Maintaining the line of the hip, take hold of the calf of the raised leg and straighten up to the ceiling.
- Alternate legs.

Cues to exercise

Work on developing strong straight legs. Create opposite motion, pressing your legs into your arms.

Breathing pattern

Breathe in to prepare. Breathe out as you pull the leg up. Breathe in as you change legs.

Checkpoints

- Keep an open chest and shoulder down position by not overreaching up the leg.
- Maintain a straight leg.

Pitfalls

- Losing control of the neutral spine.
- Placing stress on the lower spine. (The exercise is too challenging at this stage.)
- Losing head control, and allowing the chin to poke forward.

Muscle focus

Abdominals. Hamstrings. Hip flexors. Deep neck flexors.

DOUBLE STRAIGHT LEG STRETCH

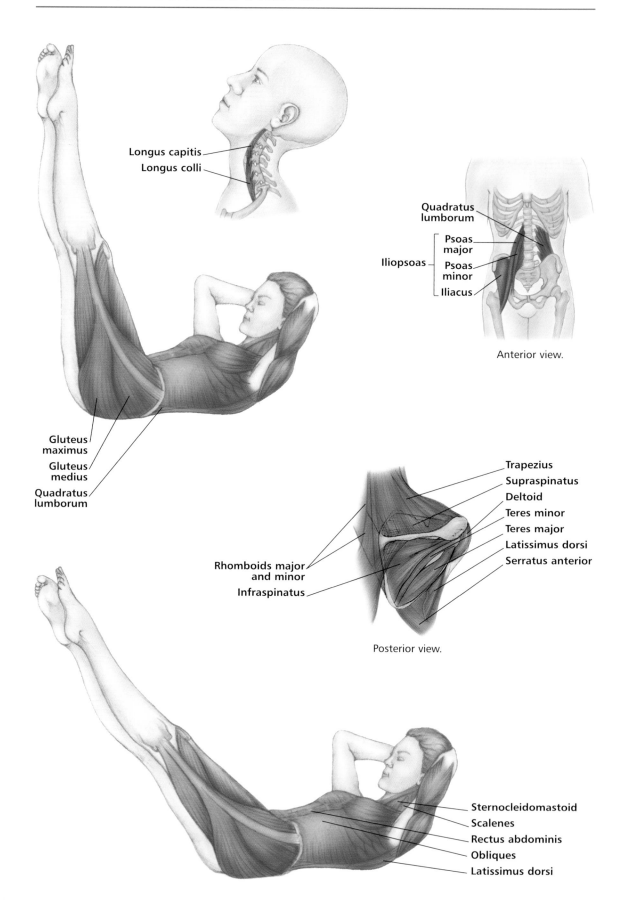

Longus capitis
Longus colli

Quadratus lumborum

Iliopsoas
- Psoas major
- Psoas minor
- Iliacus

Anterior view.

Gluteus maximus
Gluteus medius
Quadratus lumborum

Trapezius
Supraspinatus
Deltoid
Teres minor
Teres major
Latissimus dorsi
Serratus anterior

Rhomboids major and minor
Infraspinatus

Posterior view.

Sternocleidomastoid
Scalenes
Rectus abdominis
Obliques
Latissimus dorsi

Objectives of exercise
Strengthen abdominals. Enhance trunk stability. Develop coordination and flowing movement.

Exercise description
- Lie on your back and interlace your hands behind your head, with your legs straight into the air in the Pilates leg position.
- Curl up on the out breath, to a point where the shoulder blades are off the floor.
- Maintain a wide elbow position.
- Control through the breathing pattern.
- Lower the legs to a point that allows the lower back to be maintained on the mat.
- Raise the legs to the starting position.

Cue to exercise
To help the leg lift phase, think imprinting of the lower back into the mat.

Breathing pattern
Breathe in to prepare; raise your leg to return. Breathe out and lower your legs.

Checkpoints
- Keep your lower back flat on the floor. Control through the core muscle groups.
- The lower the legs, the more abdominal work. Work in a small range initially, but build the range as strength develops.
- Use your inner thighs and gluteal muscles to wrap around and control the leg lowering.

Pitfalls
- Shoulder rolling forward during curl up.
- Straining through the movement; work in the control zone of your abdominals.
- Losing control in the abdominals; bulging in the abdominals.
- Allowing your head to poke forward. Keep the head lengthened through the hands.

Muscle focus
Abdominals. Hip flexors. Deep neck flexors.

CRISS-CROSS

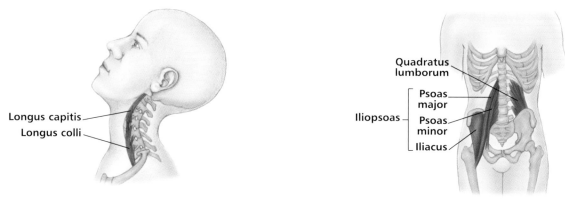

Longus capitis
Longus colli

Quadratus lumborum
Iliopsoas — Psoas major
Psoas minor
Iliacus

Anterior view.

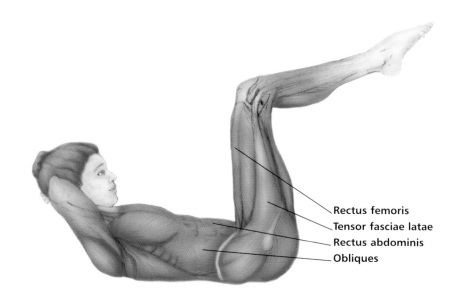

Rectus femoris
Tensor fasciae latae
Rectus abdominis
Obliques

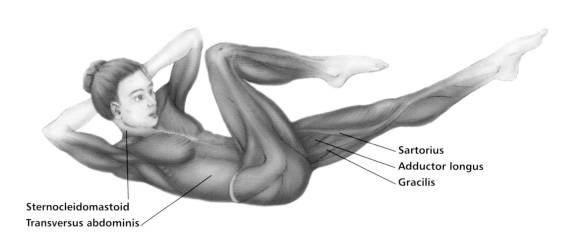

Sartorius
Adductor longus
Gracilis

Sternocleidomastoid
Transversus abdominis

Objectives of exercise

Work the oblique muscle groups. Enhance rotational control through the spine. Develop pelvic stability and trunk rotation. Reinforce the concept of thoracic breathing.

Exercise description

- Lie on the floor with your knees up, and feet hip-width apart. Your hands should be behind your head, elbows open.
- Engage your lower abdominal muscles and draw up your right shoulder toward your opposite knee. Your chest should be aimed toward your knee. Keep your elbows open.
- Continue the curl-up until both shoulder blades are off the floor.
- Hold this position, and then lower your upper body slowly to the floor.
- Repeat on the opposite side.

Cues to exercise

Keep the shoulder blades off the floor throughout the exercise. Keep the elbows open.

Breathing pattern

Breathe out during the curl up. Breathe in on the curl down.

Checkpoints

- Don't lead the movement with your elbow; lead through the front of the shoulder, maintaining the connection through your shoulder blades.
- Don't place any strain on your neck by pulling it forward.
- Don't allow your trunk or pelvis to move toward your head as you curl up.
- Extend and bend the leg in line with the hips.
- Keep the elbows wide and stable.
- Rotate from the waist and avoid moving side-flexion.

Pitfalls

- Losing the curl-up as you rotate through the spine.
- Losing the neutral spine during the exercise.

Muscle focus

Obliques. Quadratus lumborum. Lower abdominals. Hip flexors. Deep neck flexors.

SPINE STRETCH FORWARD

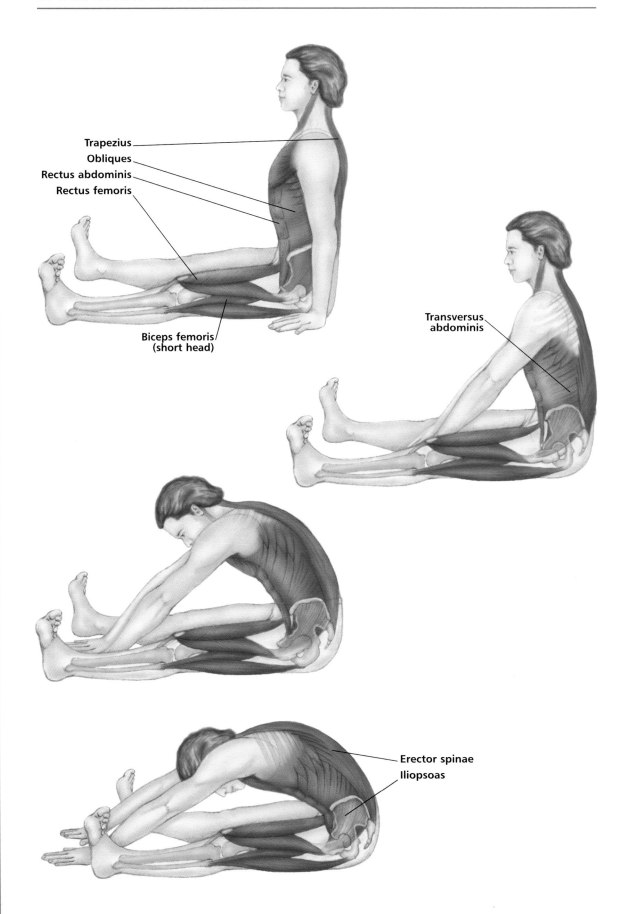

Trapezius

Obliques

Rectus abdominis

Rectus femoris

Biceps femoris
(short head)

Transversus
abdominis

Erector spinae

Iliopsoas

Objectives of exercise
Stretching the spine and back extensors.

Exercise description
- In long sitting (sitting with your legs in parallel out in front of you) with the legs wide apart, draw the toes upward and backward.
- Rest the palms forward (eventually resting palms flat on the mat). Then with the arms outstretched, and the palms low toward the floor, begin reaching forward whilst keeping the base of the spine on the mat.

Cues to exercise
Sit up and out of your hips while pulling your lower abdominals in as you curl forward. Start and create a C-curve in the spine, first with the lumbar, then the thoracic, and then the cervical spine.

Breathing pattern
Breathe out on your way down, concentrating on the end of the breath at the furthest point of your stretch.

Checkpoints
- Don't hunch your shoulders or let them rise as you reach forward.
- Maintain the lower abdominals throughout the stretch.
- Force all the air from the lungs while reaching and curling.

Pitfalls
- Slumping forward into the stretch.
- Losing abdominal contraction during the stretch.
- Forcing the movement.

Muscle focus
Lower abdominals. Hamstrings. Back extensors. Psoas. Hip flexors.

OPEN LEG ROCKER

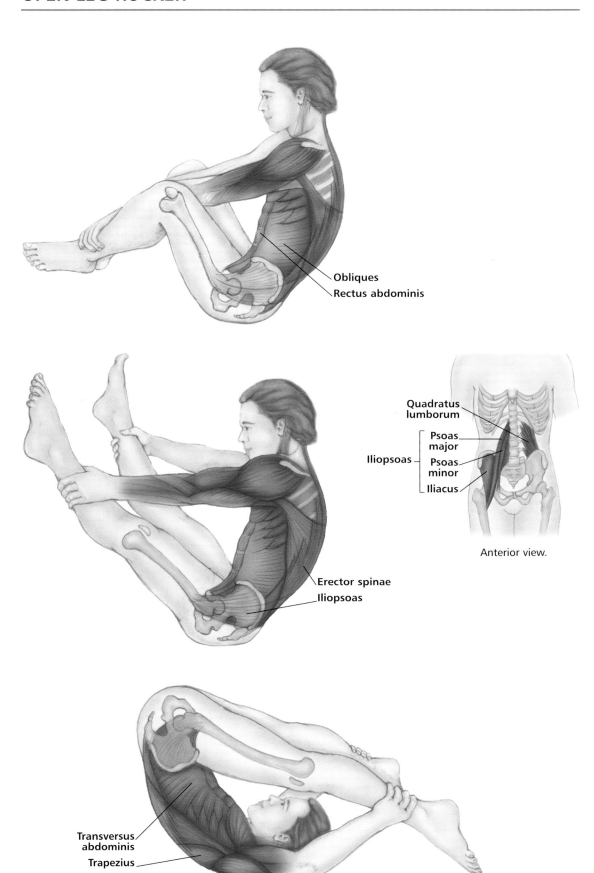

Obliques
Rectus abdominis

Quadratus lumborum

Iliopsoas {
Psoas major
Psoas minor
Iliacus

Anterior view.

Erector spinae
Iliopsoas

Transversus abdominis
Trapezius

Objectives of exercise
Improve spinal mobility. Improve balance. Enhance trunk stability. Stretch the hamstrings and spine.

Exercise description
- Sit in a V-position, balanced on your sit bones (bony regions located deep in gluteus) with the knees bent. The back needs to be held in a straight position.
- Taking hold of your ankles with your hands, keep the legs shoulder-width apart.
- Round the back, initiating the movement from the lumbar spine, and roll back to the shoulder, while straightening your legs.
- Roll back up, first keeping the spine round, and then extending it as you return to the starting position.
- Balance momentarily before repeating the exercise.

Cue to exercise
Roll like a ball.

Breathing pattern
Breathe in as you roll back. Breathe out in the balance position.

Checkpoints
- Maintain the shoulder stabilizers down during the exercise, with the elbows soft.
- Maintain deep abdominal contraction throughout the movement.
- Maintain a flat back at the start position.

Pitfalls
- Rolling too far onto your neck.
- Allowing the legs to collapse in toward you as you roll back.

Muscle focus
Abdominals. Back extensors. Iliopsoas.

DOUBLE LEG CIRCLES (CORK SCREW)

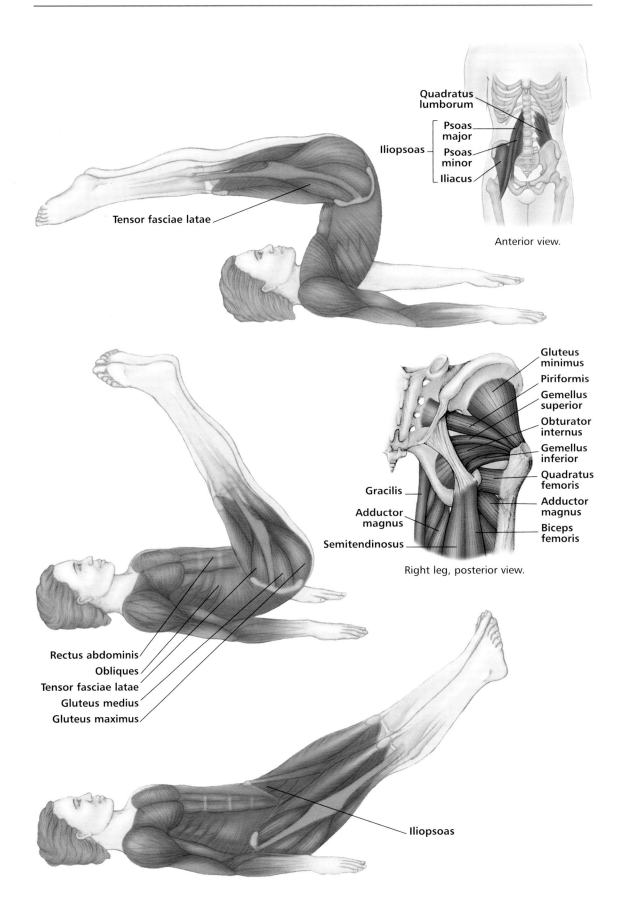

Quadratus
lumborum

Iliopsoas
- Psoas major
- Psoas minor
- Iliacus

Tensor fasciae latae

Anterior view.

Gluteus minimus
Piriformis
Gemellus superior
Obturator internus
Gemellus inferior
Quadratus femoris
Adductor magnus
Biceps femoris

Gracilis
Adductor magnus
Semitendinosus

Right leg, posterior view.

Rectus abdominis
Obliques
Tensor fasciae latae
Gluteus medius
Gluteus maximus

Iliopsoas

Objectives of exercise
Strengthen abdominals. Challenge trunk stability. Stretch the spine.

Exercise description
- Anchor down your spine (neck to base) onto the mat. Your hands should be by your side, pressing the palms into the mat for stability. Connect your shoulder blades back and down. Maintain a strong trunk.
- Raise your legs up to the ceiling, lengthening the legs away from the hips, and keep the knees and ankles together.
- Circle your legs, leading with your toes, allowing your hips to come off the mat slightly. Keep your knees and ankles together continuously.
- Complete the circle to the start position with the feet raised to the ceiling.

Cues to exercise
Don't let your pelvis go off centre during the exercise. Focus on the movement in the waist region. Bend your knees if required to reduce the strain on the hip flexors and lower back.

Breathing pattern
Breathe in as you circle your legs down. Breathe out as you circle your legs up.

Checkpoints
- Maintain pressure through the arms into the mat.
- Raising the hips from the floor will increase the challenge of the exercise.
- No stomach bulging throughout the exercise.
- Maintain connection through the thighs.
- Take care not to lose alignment through the legs during the exercise.

Pitfalls
- Allowing the back or neck to arch as the weight of the legs circle down.
- Allowing the neck to become tense.
- Hunching the shoulders.
- Allowing the legs to bend or separate during the exercise.
- Undertaking too large a circle with the feet, too quickly, and without sufficient abdominal control or strength.

Muscle focus
Iliopsoas. Rectus abdominis. Obliques. Quadratus lumborum. Hip rotators. TFL. Gluteals. Piriformis.

SAW

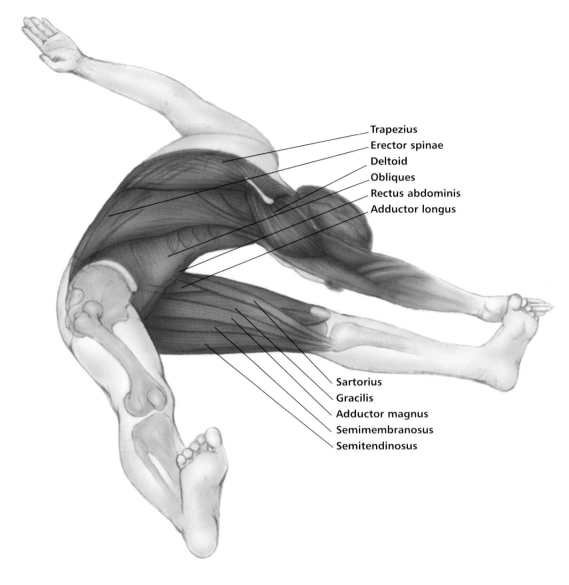

Trapezius
Erector spinae
Deltoid
Obliques
Rectus abdominis
Adductor longus

Sartorius
Gracilis
Adductor magnus
Semimembranosus
Semitendinosus

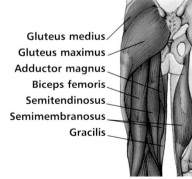

Gluteus medius
Gluteus maximus
Adductor magnus
Biceps femoris
Semitendinosus
Semimembranosus
Gracilis

Posterior view.

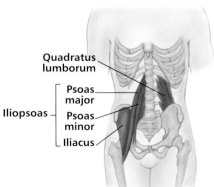

Quadratus
lumborum
Psoas
major
Iliopsoas —
Psoas
minor
Iliacus

Anterior view.

Objectives of exercise

Improve the length of the hamstrings and adductors. Develop strength of the back extensors. Enhance control into the oblique abdominal muscles. Help train spinal rotation.

Exercise description

- Sit on your sit bones (bony regions, located deep in gluteus) with your legs spread, wider than shoulder-width apart. Legs straight. Feet flexed. Arms out to the side in a T-position.
- Rotate your spine through the trunk to one side as far as possible, then bend forward and downward as far as possible, keeping your sit bones evenly balanced on the mat. Keep the arms extended in line with the shoulders and then rest diagonally and centrally on the opposite leg.
- Repeat the movement on the opposite side.

Cues to exercise

Keep the back extensors engaged when reaching forward. Keep the feet pulled up.

Breathing pattern

Breathe in to sit taller on the sit bones. Breathe out as you fold forward. Breathe in on your return to the start position.

Checkpoints

- Maintain even weight on your sit bones throughout the exercise.
- Keep the legs straight. Push out through your heels.
- On the return movement, visualise a sliding back onto a pole, sitting up out of your hips, but don't arch your back.
- Keep your lower abdominals glued to your spine.
- Ensure that the reaching hand does not drop below the level of your toes.

Pitfalls

- Rounding your back as you reach out of the sit bones, and losing spine extension.
- Maintain the spine as a whole, rather than as segments.
- Reaching for the foot, or rotating into it.
- Forcing the stretch; maintain control throughout the movement.

Muscle focus

Hamstrings. Adductors. Back extensors. Quadratus lumborum. Spinal rotators and lateral flexors (erector spinae).

SWAN DIVE

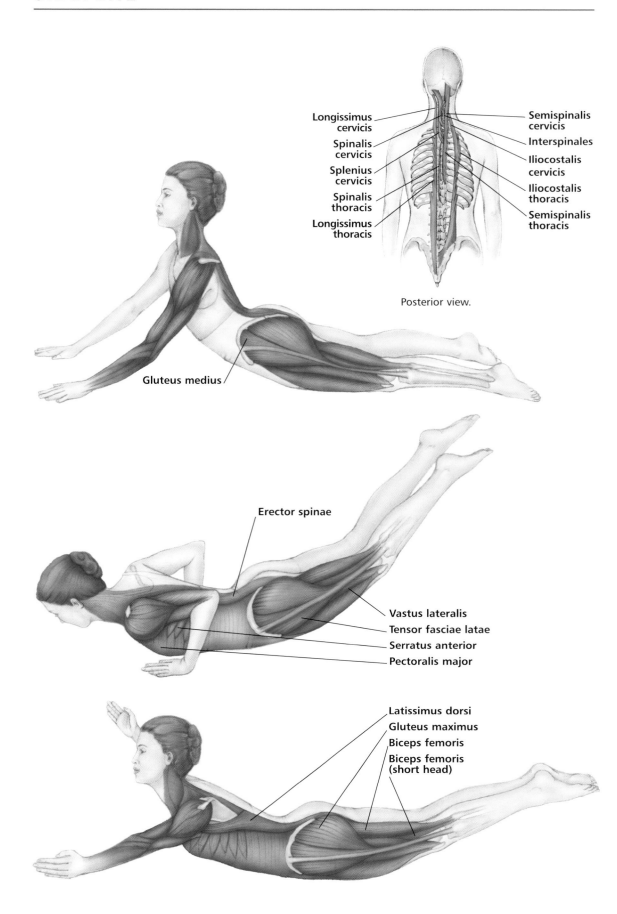

Longissimus cervicis

Spinalis cervicis

Splenius cervicis

Spinalis thoracis

Longissimus thoracis

Semispinalis cervicis

Interspinales

Iliocostalis cervicis

Iliocostalis thoracis

Semispinalis thoracis

Posterior view.

Gluteus medius

Erector spinae

Vastus lateralis

Tensor fasciae latae

Serratus anterior

Pectoralis major

Latissimus dorsi

Gluteus maximus

Biceps femoris

Biceps femoris (short head)

Objectives of exercise

Strengthen the back extensors, hamstrings and gluteals. Stretch the chest, abdominals and hip flexors. Control of spinal extension.

Exercise description

- Lie flat on your stomach with your legs stretched straight and your toes softly pointed.
- Put your palms flat on the mat, directly under your shoulders.
- Stretch your feet out further, pushing out from your hips through your toes, lifting your feet slightly off the mat.
- At the same time, straighten your arms, lifting your torso from the mat.
- Bend your arms and let yourself rock forward.

Progression

- As you rock forward, extend your arms smoothly in front of you and outward to the sides, palms up.

Cues to exercise

Concentrate on stretching as much as you can. Build up the straightening of your arms as you build your stretch. Imagine the chest bone is the rim of a wheel as you rock.

Breathing pattern

Breathe in on the way up. Breathe out on the way down.

Checkpoints

- Pinch your buttocks tight.
- Don't let your rib cage and chest sink down.
- Don't let your shoulders hunch up.
- Lengthen through your neck (chin high).
- Reach out of your lower back with your legs.
- Don't collapse on your way down.
- Maintain the arc shape of the spine throughout the movement.

Pitfall

- Need to maintain movement smoothly throughout the exercise.

Muscle focus

Gluteals. Back extensors. Hamstrings. Pectorals. Abdominals. Hip flexors.

SINGLE LEG KICK

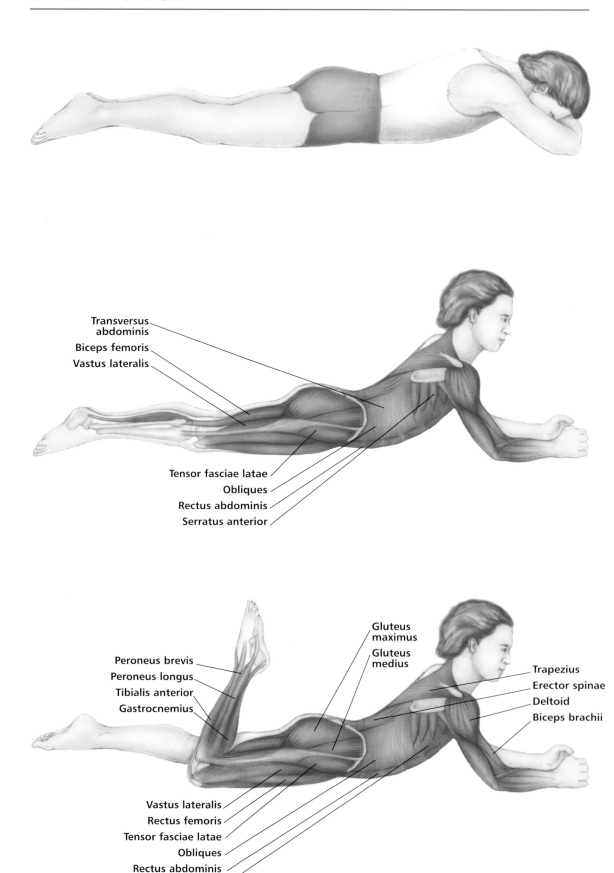

Transversus abdominis
Biceps femoris
Vastus lateralis

Tensor fasciae latae
Obliques
Rectus abdominis
Serratus anterior

Gluteus maximus
Gluteus medius

Trapezius
Erector spinae
Deltoid
Biceps brachii

Peroneus brevis
Peroneus longus
Tibialis anterior
Gastrocnemius

Vastus lateralis
Rectus femoris
Tensor fasciae latae
Obliques
Rectus abdominis
Pectoralis major

Objectives of exercise

Establish control of the knee flexors and hip extensors. Strengthen the middle and upper back extensors. This is a dynamic exercise, challenging coordination and rhythm.

Exercise description

- Lie flat on your stomach, with your legs parallel, and toes pointed.
- Place the elbows directly under the shoulders with your hands in line with the elbows.
- Make a fist with your hands.
- Maintain the length through the extended spine, anchoring the body on the fists, forearms, and the line across your hips. Maintain an open chest.
- Whilst maintaining your anchored position, briskly kick one heel toward your buttock, twice; emphasise kick, kick.
- Then stretch the leg out, and repeat the movement on the opposite side.
- Maintain control through the extended trunk.

Cues to exercise

Keep the deep abdominals lifted throughout, which helps in the protection of the lower back. Keep your focus forward and back of the neck long. Maintain this sphinx position stable. Push through the elbows.

Breathing pattern

Breathe in on the left leg. Breathe out on the right leg.

Checkpoints

- Avoid any movement in the trunk.
- Keep the arms active throughout the exercise, anchoring down in order to keep the upper chest lifted.
- Tighten the buttocks to aid control of the movement.
- Keep your head up and mouth closed.
- Keep the kicks sharp.
- Coordinate so that the legs pass each other when you alternate, keeping one foot all the way back in position before you start kicking the opposite leg.

Pitfalls

- Collapsing into the chest; there is a need to maintain an open chest line.
- Losing length in the trunk, and sagging into the back.
- Allowing the feet to touch the mat.

Muscle focus

Hip extensors. Hamstrings. Pectorals. Gluteals. Back extensors. Quadriceps. Abdominals.

DOUBLE LEG KICK

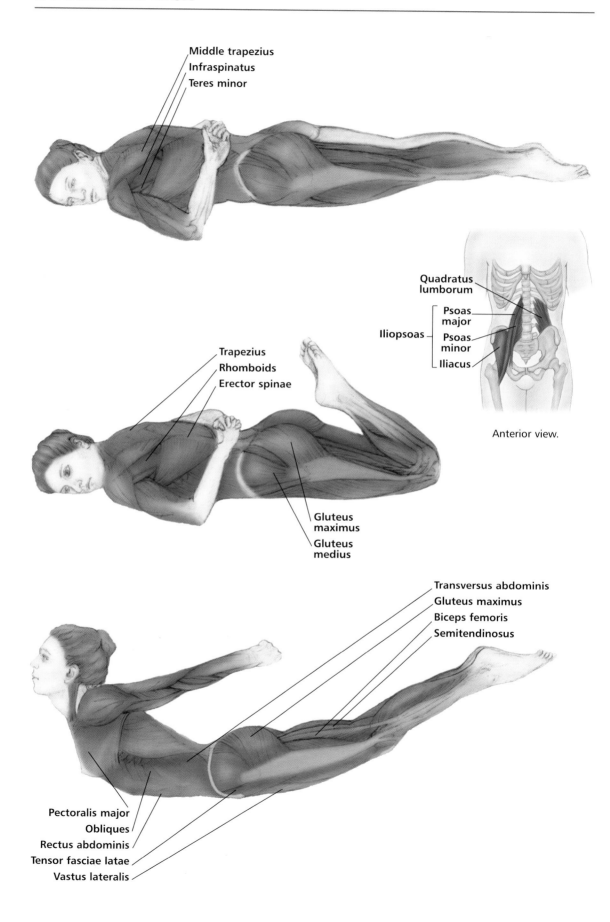

Middle trapezius
Infraspinatus
Teres minor

Quadratus lumborum
Psoas major
Iliopsoas
Psoas minor
Iliacus

Anterior view.

Trapezius
Rhomboids
Erector spinae

Gluteus maximus
Gluteus medius

Transversus abdominis
Gluteus maximus
Biceps femoris
Semitendinosus

Pectoralis major
Obliques
Rectus abdominis
Tensor fasciae latae
Vastus lateralis

Objectives of exercise

Strengthen the back extensors. Enhance control into the hamstrings. Opening the chest enhances movement throughout the thoracic spine.

Exercise description

- Lie on your stomach, head turned to the side, legs together, and feet pointed.
- Clasp your hands behind your back, placing them as high up your spine as you can.
- Keep your elbows wide, and touching the mat.
- Bend both knees and kick them toward your bottom three times, with both feet, keeping the knees and feet together. Brisk and rapid kicks.
- After three kicks, stretch your clamped hands out behind you, reaching down your back, and simultaneously, raise your legs off the mat.
- Maintain this position, and reach upward with your chin toward the ceiling.
- Release the hold, return to the mat, turning your head to the opposite side.

Cues to exercise

Maintain a stable pelvis. Maintain deep abdominals, pubic bone pressed into the mat and contract your gluteals throughout.

Breathing pattern

Breathe out and kick, kick, kick. Breathe in as you stretch out long. Breathe out and return to the start position.

Checkpoints

- Maintain strong abdominals to prevent collapsing into the spine during the kicks.
- Aim to hold the elbows as low as possible whilst kicking.
- Maintain good abdominal and gluteal contraction whilst you lift your legs.
- Emphasise lengthening the spine rather than height gained while extending.
- Maintain an open chest and front of shoulders, with the elbows wide.

Pitfalls

- Weak knee kicks (need to be strong). Aim for heels to bottom.
- Pinching shoulder blades together and drawing the shoulders down.
- Losing length in your neck.
- Collapsing when returning to the mat – maintain control.

Muscle focus

Lumbar extensors. Gluteals. Hamstrings. Rhomboids. Middle trapezius. Abdominals. Hip flexors. Pectorals. Infraspinatus. Teres minor.

NECK PULL

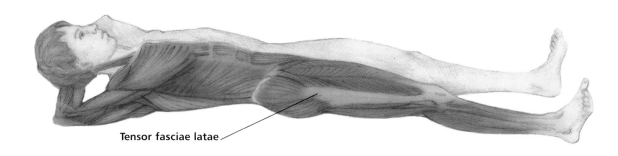

Tensor fasciae latae

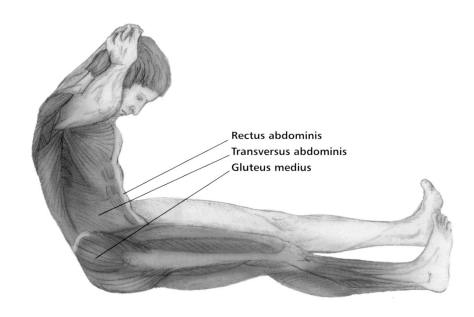

Rectus abdominis
Transversus abdominis
Gluteus medius

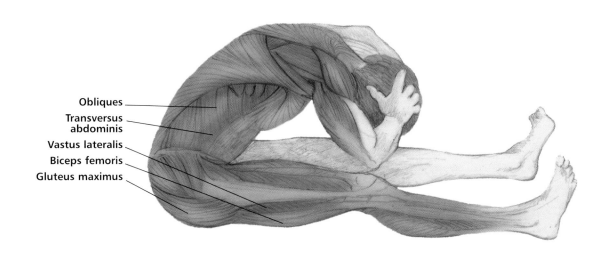

Obliques
Transversus abdominis
Vastus lateralis
Biceps femoris
Gluteus maximus

Objectives of exercise

Stretch the spine. Strengthen the trunk flexors (hip flexors, abdominals). Teach articulation of the spine. Improve length in the hamstrings.

Exercise description
- Lie flat with the pelvis in neutral, feet hip-width apart, fingers interlaced with the hands behind the head, and elbows wide.
- Nodding through the back of the neck, lift the head, slowly rolling the spine off the mat.
- Curl through the movement as the spine coils from the mat.
- Roll up until the shoulders are directly over the hips.
- Place your hands at your side.
- Initiate a smooth roll back through the spine, back to the mat until you are lying flat.

Cues to exercise

Engage the abdominals before you start to lift your head. Elbows open. Press your heels into the mat to cue the hamstrings. Use the imprinting concept to assist engagement of the hip extensors.

Breathing pattern
Breathe in as you curl up and then out to get yourself curled up as tightly as possible. Breathe in as you sit up. Breathe out on the way down.

Checkpoints
- Don't allow your shoulders to hunch up.
- Maintain the elbows in line with your ears and back during the exercise.
- Maintain a deep abdominal contraction throughout.
- Maintain a smooth, gradual curl up and down movement.
- Sit up tall, and note the vertical lift in the central trunk area.
- Flatten your ribs to the floor before rolling the shoulders off the mat.

Pitfalls
- Straining through the movement.
- Rushing the curl up action; you need to keep the movement smooth.
- Pulling on the neck, and allowing the elbows to lose the alignment with the ears.
- Hinging through a straight back rather than rolling down through the spine.

Muscle focus
Abdominals. Hip flexors. Hamstrings. Gluteals.

SCISSORS

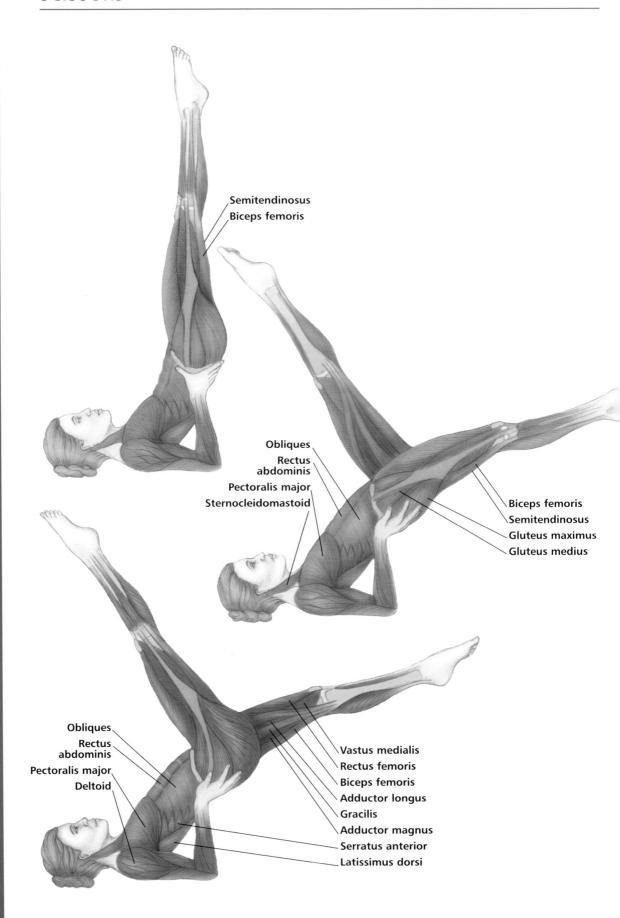

Semitendinosus
Biceps femoris

Obliques
Rectus abdominis
Pectoralis major
Sternocleidomastoid

Biceps femoris
Semitendinosus
Gluteus maximus
Gluteus medius

Obliques
Rectus abdominis
Pectoralis major
Deltoid

Vastus medialis
Rectus femoris
Biceps femoris
Adductor longus
Gracilis
Adductor magnus
Serratus anterior
Latissimus dorsi

Objectives of exercise

Enhance abdominal control. Develop hip extensor and flexor control and flexibility. Enhance stabilization through the shoulder and trunk.

Exercise description
- Lie flat on your back with your legs straight out and together.
- Stretch your neck long and press the base of your skull to the mat.
- Raise your legs to a ninety-degree angle with your body, and at the same time swing your hips up off the mat, lengthening the toes to the ceiling.
- Place your hands on your back above your hips, with the elbows on the mat directly below your hands. The higher you raise your body, the more support on your back with your hand position.
- While maintaining good control of your trunk, stretch your toes up to the ceiling, maintaining the stretch upward, and reach past your bottom with your toes on one leg, maintaining a straight leg.
- Allow the other leg to move slightly in the direction of your head to maintain your balance.
- Reverse the scissor action.

Cues to exercise

Allow the pelvis to drop heavy into the hands.

Breathing pattern
Breathe in, reaching back with one leg, and alternate with the breath out, as you reach back with the alternate leg.

Checkpoints
- Strength for the exercise comes from the shoulders and upper arms in order to maintain your centre, and not via your hands and arms. Overuse of the arms and hands will prevent smooth movement.
- Maintain deep abdominal contraction.
- Maintain control over the hips, which should remain motionless during the exercise.
- Concentrate on stretching your legs past your bottom.
- Balance the distance you move your legs, which should be kept even.
- Keep elbows parallel to each other.

Pitfalls
- Using the base of the skull as the balance control point. Balance is controlled through your abdominals and gluteals.
- Bending your knees.
- Using the arms as the main support; control comes from lengthening or use of the abdominals.
- Allowing the chin to collapse onto the chest, which will limit your ability to breathe.

Muscle focus

Upper back. Hip extensors. Hip flexors.

BICYCLE

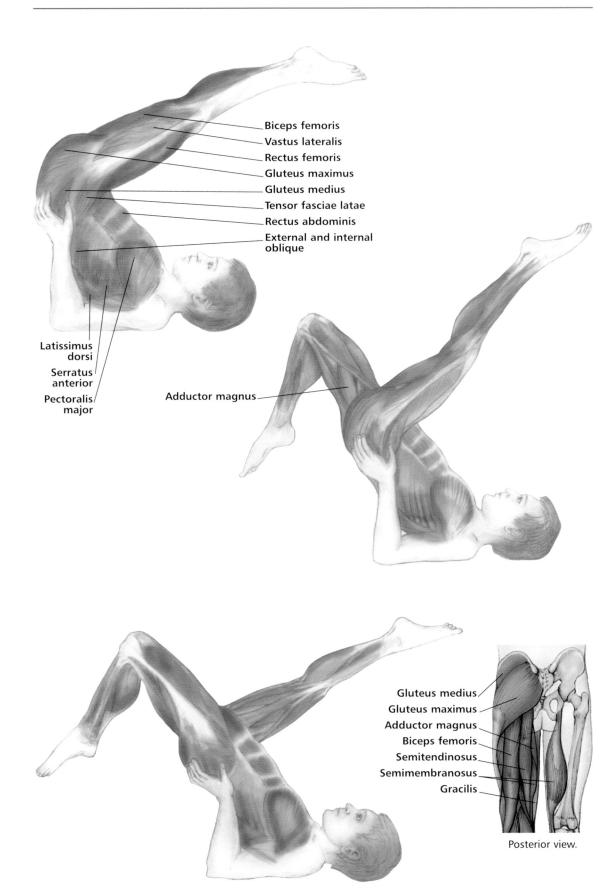

Biceps femoris
Vastus lateralis
Rectus femoris
Gluteus maximus
Gluteus medius
Tensor fasciae latae
Rectus abdominis
External and internal oblique

Latissimus dorsi
Serratus anterior
Pectoralis major

Adductor magnus

Gluteus medius
Gluteus maximus
Adductor magnus
Biceps femoris
Semitendinosus
Semimembranosus
Gracilis

Posterior view.

Objectives of exercise
Improve hip flexor control. Improve flexibility in the hips.

Exercise description
- Lie flat on your back with your legs straight out and together.
- Stretch your neck long and press the base of your skull to the mat.
- Raise your legs to a ninety-degree angle with your body, and at the same time, swing your hips up off the mat, lengthening the toes to the ceiling.
- Place your hands on your back, above your hips, and your elbows on the mat directly below your hands. The higher you raise your body, the more support on your back with your hand position.
- Stretch your toes toward the ceiling.
- Maintain length in one leg, bend the other leg and reach your toes past your bottom.
- Keep the leg moving in an arc; imagine reaching out along a wall and back along the floor, and straighten the leg to point the foot at the ceiling.
- Maintain length upward with a stationary leg (use as a counter balance), by small movement toward your head.
- When the leg returns to the start position, repeat the pattern with the opposite leg.

Cues to exercise
Control the trunk with coordinated movement; reach for the ceiling with one foot as the other sweeps along the floor.

Breathing pattern
Breathe in reaching for the floor. Alternate with the out breath for the other leg.

Checkpoints
- It is important to maintain control in your trunk; over reliance on your hands and arms will limit the movement properly.
- Reach out past your bottom for the wall behind you, and then for the floor, with a coordinated foot action.
- Coordinate movement, so that both feet are moving smoothly at the same time.
- Maintain a straight spine.

Pitfalls
- Allowing your knees to drop toward your face; maintain height.
- Allowing the pelvis to fall heavily into your hands.

Muscle focus
Hip extensors. Upper trunk.

SHOULDER BRIDGE

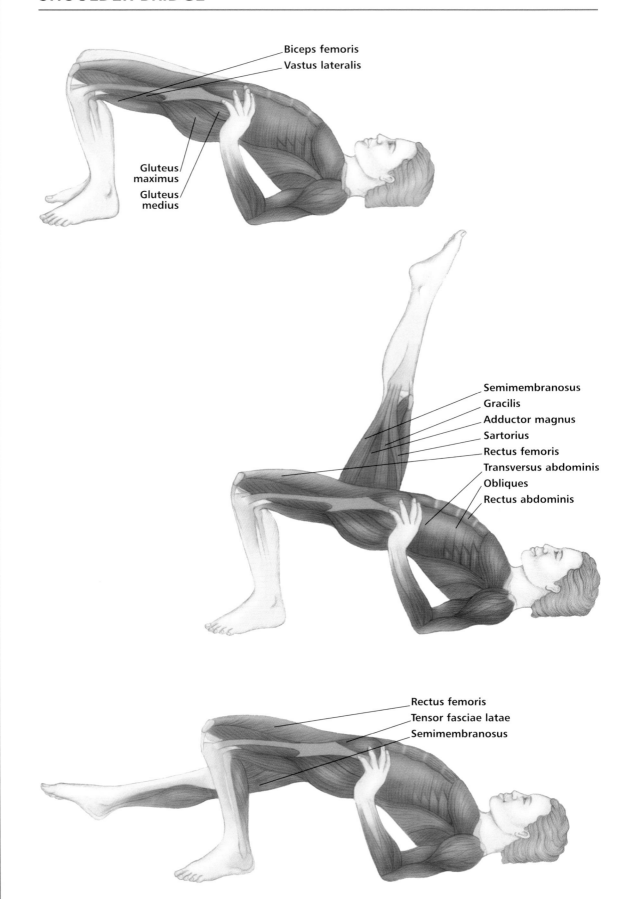

Biceps femoris
Vastus lateralis
Gluteus maximus
Gluteus medius

Semimembranosus
Gracilis
Adductor magnus
Sartorius
Rectus femoris
Transversus abdominis
Obliques
Rectus abdominis

Rectus femoris
Tensor fasciae latae
Semimembranosus

Objectives of exercise
Strengthen the hip extensors. Maintain trunk extension. Lengthen the hamstrings. Improve shoulder stabilization. Teach single leg balance.

Exercise description
- Lie in a neutral position, lift your hips from the mat, and support them with your hands under each hip bone.
- While maintaining a high hip position, softly point one leg through the toes; stretch the leg long from the hip.
- Kick the leg up as high as is comfortable, and maintain length.
- At the top of your range, flex the foot, and then slowly lower the leg, pushing the heel away to just above the floor.
- Softly point the toe and repeat for three kicks, then change onto the opposite leg.

Cues to exercise
Maintain relaxed shoulders. Lengthening the leg as you stretch it up and down.

Breathing pattern
Breathe in as your leg kicks up. Breathe out as you lower your leg.

Checkpoints
- Keep your pelvis high off the mat.
- Maintain tight muscle contraction in your gluteals.
- Stretch your leg long out of your hips.
- Maintain control of the hip height and prevent movement. Maintain connection of the shoulder and trunk–pelvis (draw the shoulder down).
- Foot needs to be under the knee.
- As the leg lowers, do not allow the leg to roll out.

Pitfalls
- Hip movement.
- Inability to control bridge position.
- Twisting through the trunk. You need to maintain the trunk and pelvis square.
- Loss of control from the arm support. The wrist needs to be in line with the elbows.
- Losing gluteal contraction during the exercise.

Muscle focus
Hip flexors. Hamstrings. Gluteals. Abdominals. Hip extensors. Adductors.

SPINE TWIST

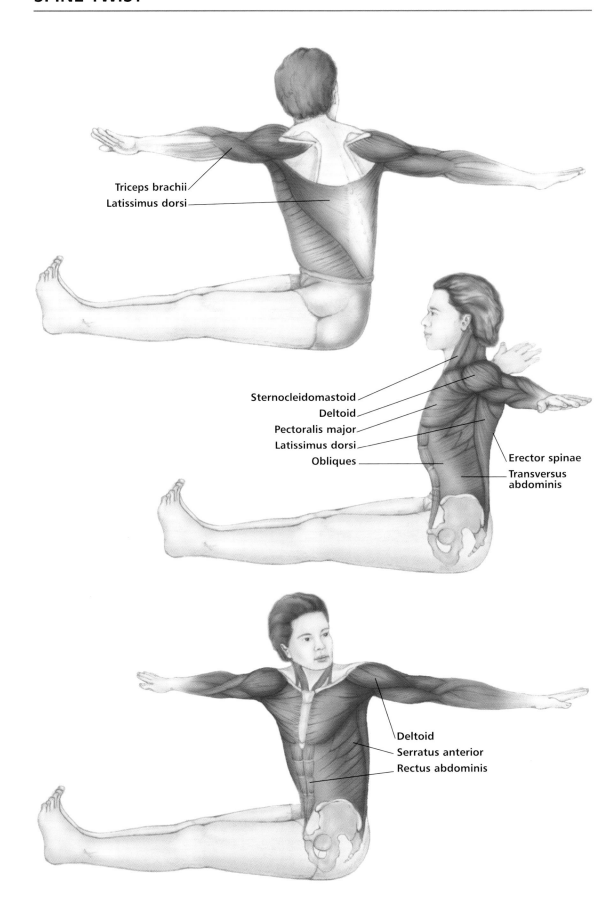

Triceps brachii
Latissimus dorsi

Sternocleidomastoid
Deltoid
Pectoralis major
Latissimus dorsi
Obliques

Erector spinae
Transversus abdominis

Deltoid
Serratus anterior
Rectus abdominis

Objectives of exercise

Strengthen the obliques, abdominals and back extensors. Enhance spinal mobility. Enhance postural control in sitting.

Exercise description
- Sit straight with your legs together and parallel. Feet flexed.
- Reach the arms out to the side, palms facing down.
- Lengthen the spine; sit up and out of your hips.
- Start the twist through the head and then rotate through the spine.
- At the end of the range, hold the position for a moment, and then rotate back to the starting position.
- Repeat in the opposite direction.

Cues to exercise

Push the heels away from you in sitting, and feel the stretch. As you turn, imagine sliding the spine up a pole.

Breathing pattern
Breathe in, in the neutral position. Breathe out forcefully when you twist.

Checkpoints
- Maintain deep abdominal contractions throughout the exercise.
- Carry arms with the spine; do not lead the movement through the arms.
- Ensure the pelvis remains still and square to your feet, with the legs still. Use your hip adductors.
- Keep the spine in the lengthened position throughout.

Pitfalls
- Allowing your shoulders to lift when you sit out of your hips.
- Allowing your head to tilt rather than turn.
- Allowing your arms to move out of chest line, either twisting back or leading the movement.
- Allowing the pelvis to move.
- Tight hamstrings and weak hip flexors.

Muscle focus

Abdominals. Obliques. Back extensors.

JACK KNIFE

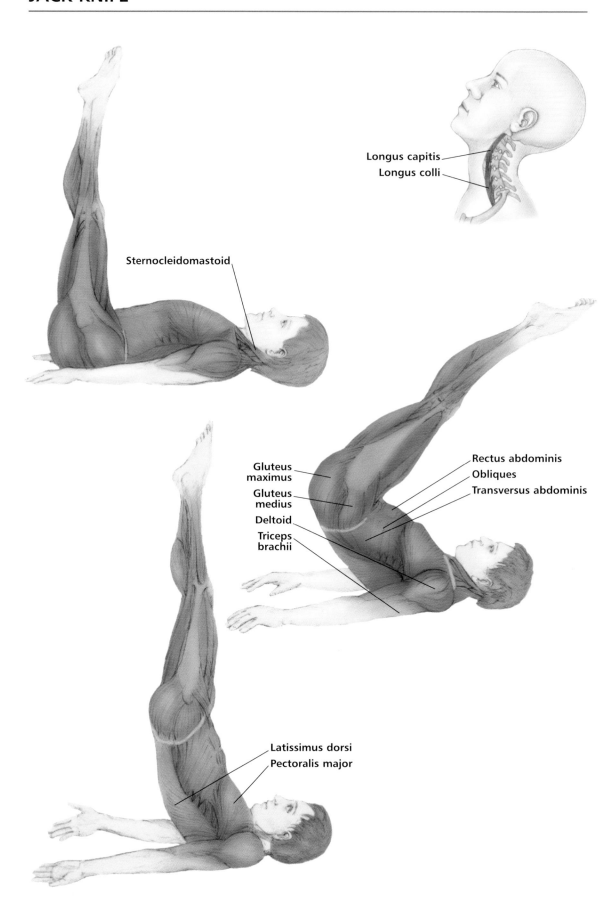

Longus capitis

Longus colli

Sternocleidomastoid

Gluteus maximus

Gluteus medius

Deltoid

Triceps brachii

Rectus abdominis

Obliques

Transversus abdominis

Latissimus dorsi

Pectoralis major

Objectives of exercise
Enhance abdominal strength and control. Strengthen hip extensors. Develop spinal articulation. Stretch the spine.

Exercise description
- Lie on your back, arms at your side, palms pressed down, and raise both legs straight above the pelvis.
- Whilst keeping the legs fully extended, toes softly pointed to the ceiling and the hips on the mat, lift your hips off the mat and let your legs swing toward your head. Keep the movement controlled.
- Continue reaching upward with your legs until your legs create a forty-five degree angle with the mat.
- While in the raised position, bring the leg up toward the ceiling.
- From this raised position, gradually roll down your back to the mat, maintaining control. Your legs should smoothly jack knife through the movement as they make their way down, going back to forty-five degrees over your head as they return back to the mat.

Cues to exercise
Focus on lifting and lengthening your legs away from your pelvis to maintain control through the spine. In the jack knife position, keep open hips to help activate control in the hip extensors. Use breathing pattern to help control the flow of the movement.

Breathing pattern
Breathe in on the way up. Breathe out on the way down.

Checkpoints
- Only move your weight so that you feel in your shoulder blades, and not beyond.
- Perform the jack knife as smoothly as possible, and avoid jerky movements.

Pitfalls
- Not maintaining smooth movement throughout the exercise.
- Taking the legs too far and increasing pressure on your neck. (Take weight to shoulder blade level only.)
- Keep the shoulders away from the ears, and maintain pressure down into the mat.

Muscle focus
Abdominals. Gluteals. Cervical spinal extensors. Shoulder extensors.

SIDE KICK LIFT

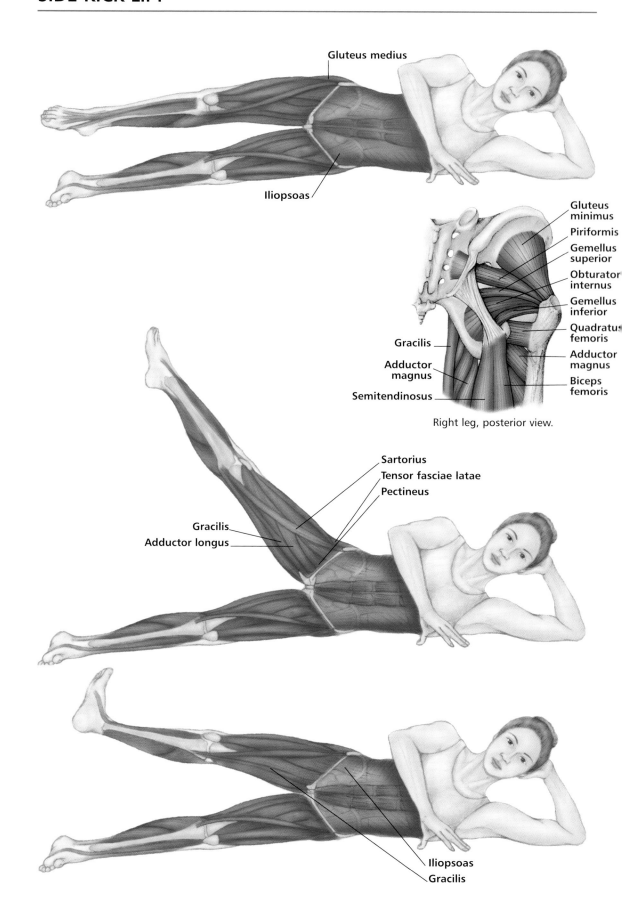

Gluteus medius

Iliopsoas

Gluteus minimus
Piriformis
Gemellus superior
Obturator internus
Gemellus inferior
Quadratus femoris
Adductor magnus
Biceps femoris

Gracilis
Adductor magnus
Semitendinosus

Right leg, posterior view.

Sartorius
Tensor fasciae latae
Pectineus
Gracilis
Adductor longus

Iliopsoas
Gracilis

Objectives of exercise
Strengthen the lateral flexors. Enhance hip adductor control.

Exercise description
- Lie on your side in a straight line, shoulder over shoulder, hip over hip, and ankles together.
- Bring both legs forwards to 45 degrees from the body line.
- Prop your head up on your arm with the elbow in line with your shoulder.
- Place the top hand behind the head, reaching the elbow toward the ceiling.
- Lift the top leg to a point level with the pelvis; the pelvis and spine remain stable.
- Sweep the top leg forward and back, hinging from the hip. At the end of the sweep forward, pull the feet up and draw the movement back through the heel.
- Repeat on the opposite side.

Cues to exercise
Lengthen through the heel.

Breathing pattern
Breathe in as you kick forward. Breathe out as you kick back.

Checkpoints
- Keep the legs parallel.
- Controlled range of motion with balanced control.
- Leg must move in isolation.

Pitfalls
- Allowing the legs to drop.
- Allowing the body to move; you need to maintain a stable spine.

Muscle focus
Hip abductors. Hip adductors. Gluteals.

SIDE-LYING LEG CIRCLES

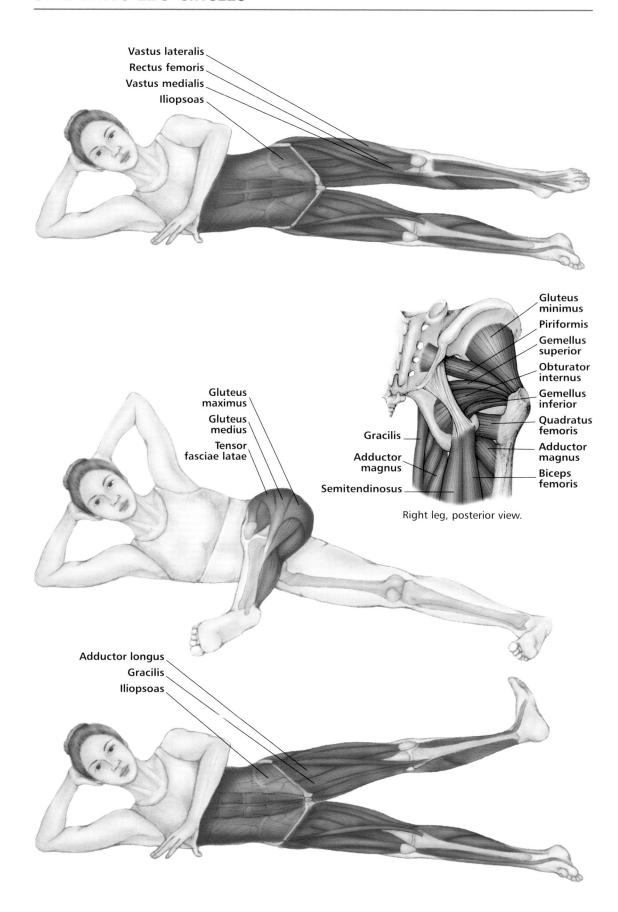

Vastus lateralis
Rectus femoris
Vastus medialis
Iliopsoas

Gluteus minimus
Piriformis
Gemellus superior
Obturator internus
Gemellus inferior
Quadratus femoris
Adductor magnus
Biceps femoris

Gracilis
Adductor magnus
Semitendinosus

Right leg, posterior view.

Gluteus maximus
Gluteus medius
Tensor fasciae latae

Adductor longus
Gracilis
Iliopsoas

Objectives of exercise
Strengthen the lateral flexors. Enhance hip adductor control.

Exercise description
- Lie on your side in a straight line, shoulder over shoulder, hip over hip, and ankles together.
- Bring both legs forward to 45 degrees from the body line.
- Prop the head up on your arm with the elbow in line with your shoulder.
- Place the top hand behind the head, reaching the elbow toward the ceiling.
- Lift the top leg to a point level with the pelvis; the pelvis and spine remain stable.
- Lengthen the leg and circle in a controlled manner.
- Hinging from the hip, draw the movement back through the heel.
- Repeat on the opposite side.

Cues to exercise
Lengthen through the heel. Control trunk stability with the size of the circle (start small, and build).

Breathing pattern
Breathe in as you circle up. Breathe out as you circle down.

Checkpoints
- Keep the legs parallel.
- Control the range of motion with balanced control.
- Move the leg in isolation.

Pitfalls
- Allowing the leg to drop.
- Allowing the body to move; you need to maintain a stable spine.

Muscle focus
Hip abductors. Hip adductors. Gluteals.

TORPEDO

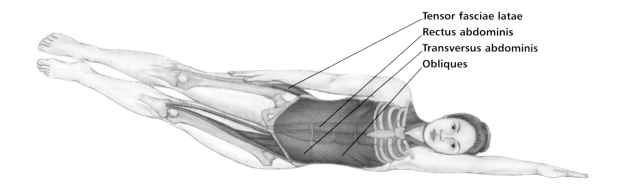

Tensor fasciae latae
Rectus abdominis
Transversus abdominis
Obliques

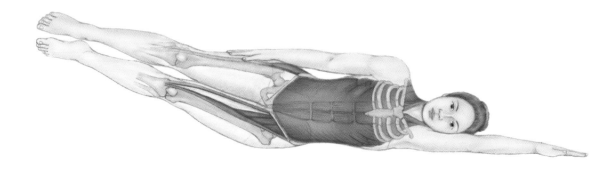

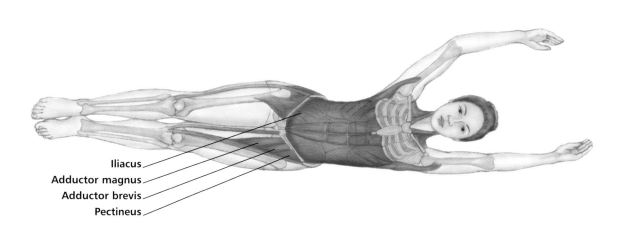

Iliacus
Adductor magnus
Adductor brevis
Pectineus

Objectives of exercise
Enhance trunk control and balance.

Exercise description
- Lie on one side with the bottom arm straight in line with the body and the head resting on it.
- The top arm is resting on your side.
- Contract your deep abdominals, lift your top leg straight off the mat, hold the raised position, and raise the bottom leg to meet it. Hold, and press them together.
- While maintaining the leg position, allow the top arm to rise above your head. Hold this position.
- Return your arm to your side, and then lower both legs back to the mat.

Cues to exercise
Stay long and lifted through the trunk.

Breathing pattern
Breathe out during the leg lift and arm movement phase. Breathe in when you return to the start position.

Checkpoints
- Avoid excessive pressure on your arms.
- Control balance through the trunk.

Pitfalls
- Losing a good quality contraction through the abdominals.
- Moving the legs backward and forward while in the balance position.

Muscle focus
Abdominals. Adductors. Abductors.

1

TEASER

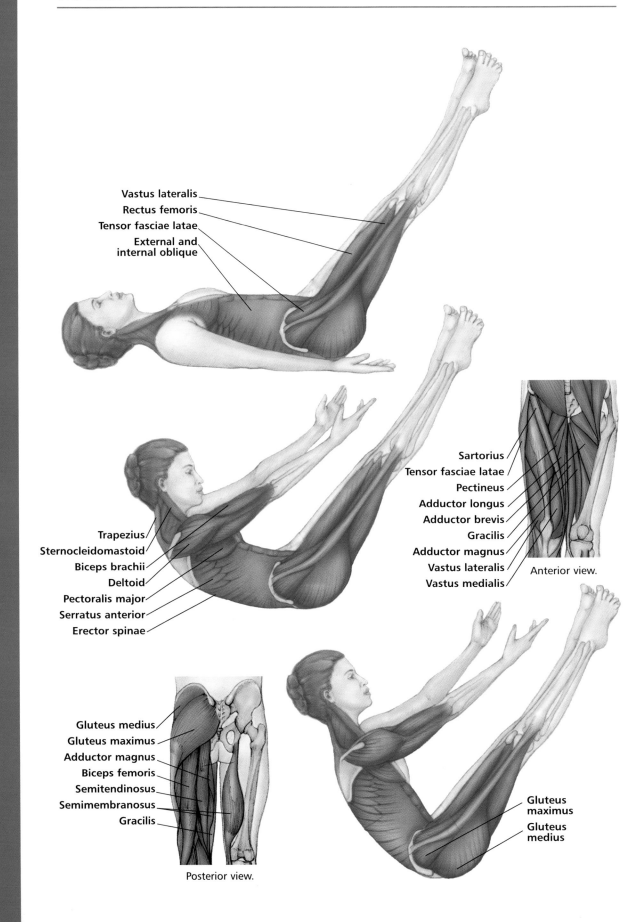

Vastus lateralis
Rectus femoris
Tensor fasciae latae
External and internal oblique

Trapezius
Sternocleidomastoid
Biceps brachii
Deltoid
Pectoralis major
Serratus anterior
Erector spinae

Sartorius
Tensor fasciae latae
Pectineus
Adductor longus
Adductor brevis
Gracilis
Adductor magnus
Vastus lateralis
Vastus medialis

Anterior view.

Gluteus medius
Gluteus maximus
Adductor magnus
Biceps femoris
Semitendinosus
Semimembranosus
Gracilis

Posterior view.

Gluteus maximus
Gluteus medius

Objectives of exercise
Strengthen flexors of the body (abdominals, hip flexors and neck flexors). Enhance control of hip flexors. Develop static balance.

Exercise description
- Lie on your back with your legs raised and extended and heels tightly together. Arms by your side with your palms up to the ceiling.
- In a controlled manner, curl up to a straight spine position, connecting shoulder to trunk and using the deep abdominals.
- Lifting your chest up and arms parallel to your shoulder. Maintain this position.
- Reverse the movement to return to the starting position.

Cues to exercise
Correct neck sequence: imagine a ball under the chin, held in position under the chin, but not squeezed. This will help the sequence in the curl-up phase. Strong contraction of the inner thigh helps leg stability.

Breathing pattern
Breathe in to prepare. Raise chest up. Breathe out, curl up, and curl down.

Checkpoints
- Strong, deep abdominal contraction.
- Control the movement (no jerky movements).
- Maintain straight legs, with toes pointed.

Pitfalls
- Allowing your shoulders to rise up.
- Allowing the heels to come apart.

Muscle focus
Quadriceps. Adductors. Gluteals. Hamstrings. Back extensors.

HIP CIRCLES

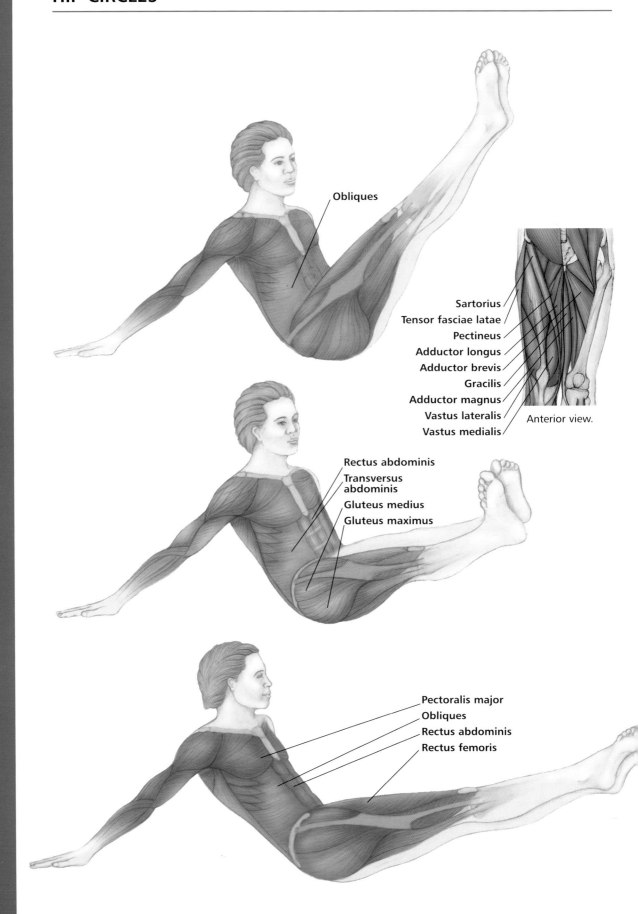

Obliques

Sartorius
Tensor fasciae latae
Pectineus
Adductor longus
Adductor brevis
Gracilis
Adductor magnus
Vastus lateralis
Vastus medialis

Anterior view.

Rectus abdominis
Transversus abdominis
Gluteus medius
Gluteus maximus

Pectoralis major
Obliques
Rectus abdominis
Rectus femoris

Objectives of exercise
Strengthen the abdominals. Enhance trunk rotation.

Exercise description
- Sit with your arms behind you, and with your palms on the mat.
- Lean back, weight bear through your hands, moving them backward to find the balance point.
- Lift both legs off the mat; your body should be forty-five degrees to the mat.
- Bend your knees to your chest.
- Straighten your legs together and keep your knees high toward the head.
- Holding this position, swing your legs in a circle, down to the right, with your feet softly pointed.
- Circle the legs, hold the top of the circle, and reverse the direction.

Cues to exercise
Control the neutral spine. Don't allow the back to extend, and control the motion.

Breathing pattern
Breathe in and swing your legs down. Breathe out as you swing your legs back up.

Checkpoints
- Keep a strong anchor of palms and base of your spine.
- Keep the size of the circle within your control, allowing a straight spine throughout.
- Arms straight.
- Keep the feet together, with knees straight.

Pitfalls
- Sinking into your shoulders and allowing the chest to sink.
- Movement through the hips (ensure control of the deep abdominals).

Muscle focus
Hip flexors. Abdominals. Chest muscles.

SWIMMING

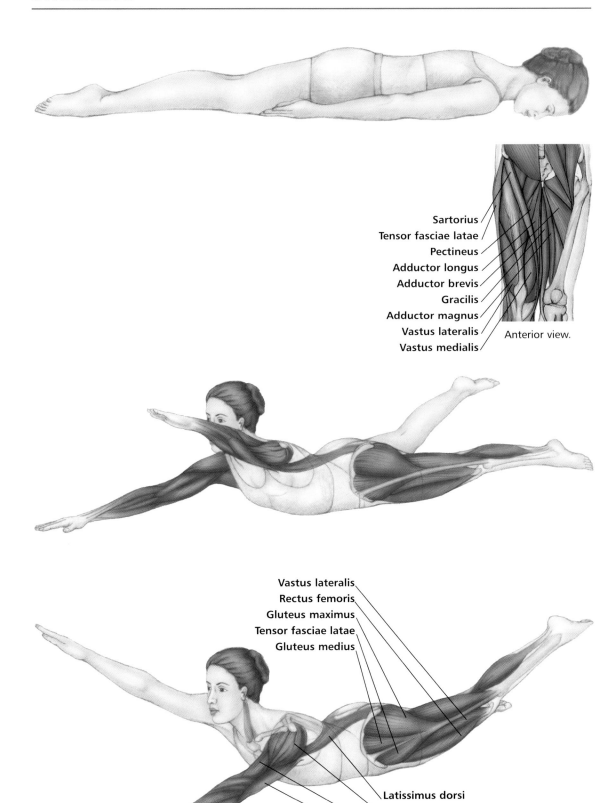

Sartorius
Tensor fasciae latae
Pectineus
Adductor longus
Adductor brevis
Gracilis
Adductor magnus
Vastus lateralis
Vastus medialis

Anterior view.

Vastus lateralis
Rectus femoris
Gluteus maximus
Tensor fasciae latae
Gluteus medius

Latissimus dorsi
Deltoid
Biceps brachii
Triceps brachii

Objectives of exercise
Strengthen the back extensors. Enhance trunk stability. Improve movement coordination. Control shoulder flexor and hip extensor control.

Exercise description
- Lie on your stomach with your arms straight in front of you, with palms down, legs slightly wider than hip-width apart, and feet turned out.
- Lift your chest, arms and legs off the mat, whilst maintaining a lengthened/stretched position.
- With controlled but fast movement (like you're beating water, but not creating big splashes) alternate lifting your arms and legs at the same speed.

Cues to exercise
Swimming action without big splashing.

Breathing pattern
Breathe in for a count of five. Breathe out for a count of five.

Checkpoints
- Maintain lengthening throughout the movement.
- Allowing the legs or arms to drop in height during the exercise.
- Pinch your bottom.
- Do not allow your shoulders to hunch up during the arm movement. Draw the shoulders down through your back.
- Maintain deep abdominals to control pelvis–trunk movement.
- Don't allow locking sensation in your lower spine.
- Breathe deeply.

Pitfalls
- Pinching in the lower back. (Ensure control of the deep abdominals throughout the exercise.)
- Losing focus on lengthening from fingertips to toes.
- Allowing the abdominals to drop into the mat during the exercise.

Muscle focus
Anterior chest muscles. Hip flexors. Back extensors.

LEG PULL FRONT

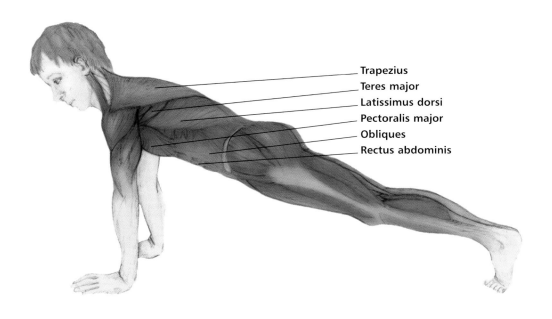

Trapezius
Teres major
Latissimus dorsi
Pectoralis major
Obliques
Rectus abdominis

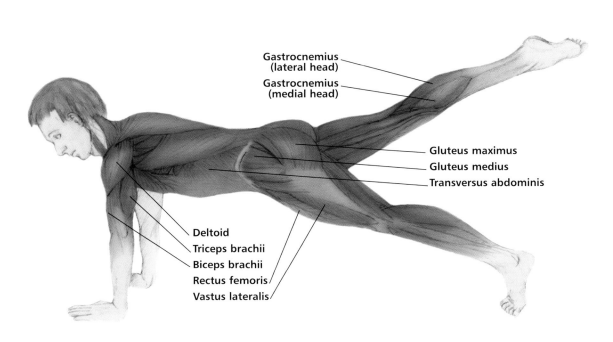

Gastrocnemius
(lateral head)
Gastrocnemius
(medial head)

Gluteus maximus
Gluteus medius
Transversus abdominis

Deltoid
Triceps brachii
Biceps brachii
Rectus femoris
Vastus lateralis

Objectives of exercise

Enhance stabilization of the trunk on the shoulder girdle. Strengthen the upper limbs. Strengthen the hip extensors and shoulder girdle.

Exercise description

- Lie in a plank position. Place your arms straight with the wrists under the shoulders.
- The legs should be straight, parallel and adducted. Weight bear through the toes.
- Make your trunk, long, thin and straight.
- Push back into your heels, and at the same time, lift one of the legs. Keep the leg straight and the hips level.
- Lower the leg.
- Repeat on the other side.

Cues to exercise

Strong centre with no movement at the hip.

Breathing pattern

Breathe in as you raise your leg. Breathe out as you lower your leg.

Checkpoints

- Contract the deep abdominals and gluteals.
- Keep the head, neck, spine, hips and leg in a straight line throughout.
- Keep the raised leg straight.
- Push hard through the heel to achieve a good stretch.

Pitfalls

- Hunching the shoulders.
- Bending up at the hip, or sinking down through the hips.

Muscle focus

Abdominals. Gluteals. Shoulder stabilizers. Quadriceps. Gastrocnemius.

LEG PULL BACK

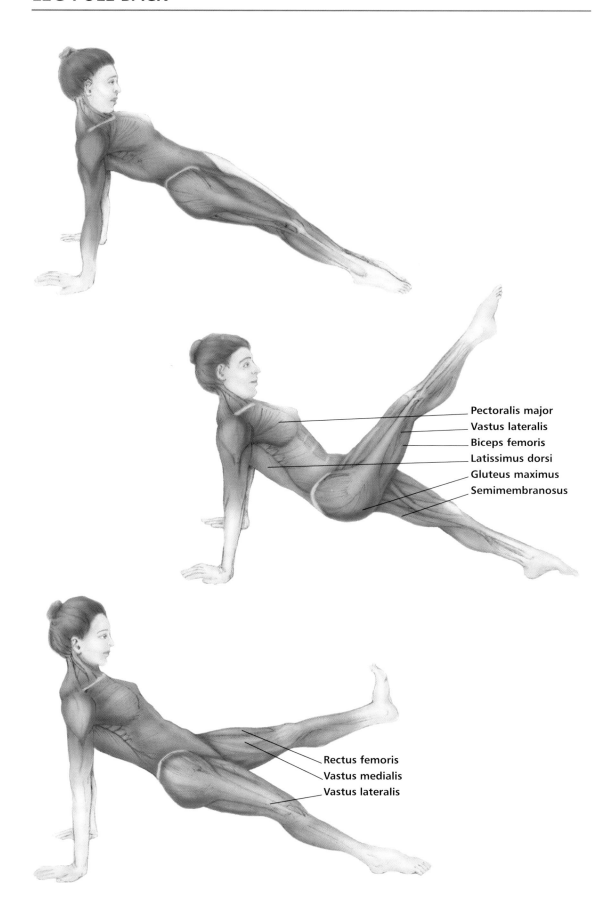

Pectoralis major
Vastus lateralis
Biceps femoris
Latissimus dorsi
Gluteus maximus
Semimembranosus

Rectus femoris
Vastus medialis
Vastus lateralis

Objectives of exercise
Muscle strengthening. Stretching the anterior chest wall.

Exercise description
- Sit upright with the legs straight in front and parallel.
- Place the hands on the mat, slightly behind the hips, with the fingers pointing forward.
- Raise your hips up from the mat, and use your deep abdominals and gluteals to a supported position on your hands and heels. Reach for the mat with your toes.
- Maintain this position with the arms straight and body stretched out from your shoulders to your toes.
- Whilst maintaining this position, with the chin on chest, kick one leg as high as you can with the toes softly pointed, reaching out from your hips. At the top of your range, flex the foot.
- Lower the leg down, pushing through the heel, maintaining a lifted hip throughout.
- Just off the mat, point the toes and kick up again.
- Repeat on the other leg.

Cues to exercise
Maintain a straight line.

Breathing pattern
Breathe in when kicking your leg up. Breathe out when lowering the leg toward the mat.

Checkpoints
- Maintain deep abdominals throughout.
- Maintain the body in a straight line.

Pitfalls
- Allowing your bottom to lower during the exercise.
- Allowing your head to sink into your shoulders.

Muscle focus
Latissimus dorsi. Hamstrings. Gluteals. Hip flexors. Quadriceps. Pectorals.

SIDE KICK KNEELING

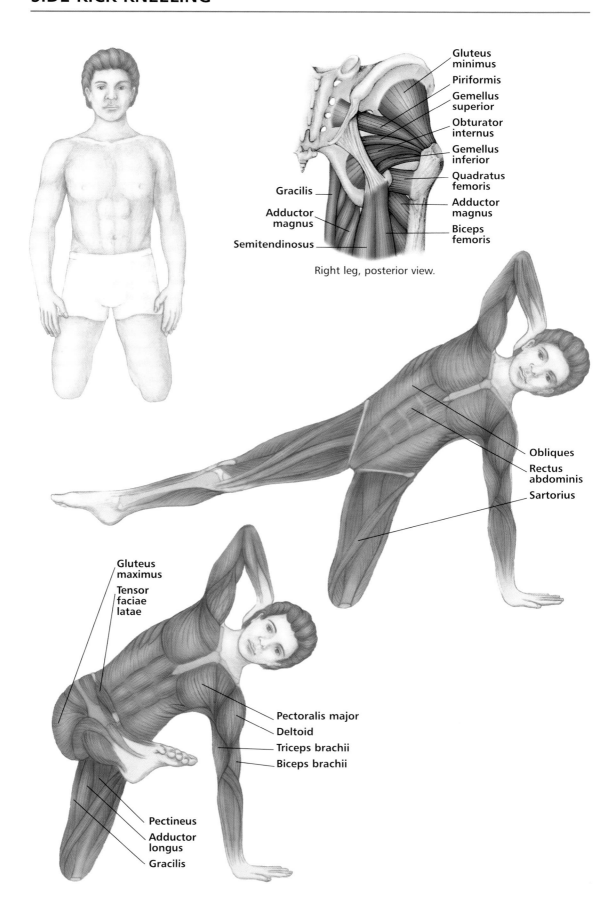

Gluteus minimus

Piriformis

Gemellus superior

Obturator internus

Gemellus inferior

Quadratus femoris

Adductor magnus

Biceps femoris

Gracilis

Adductor magnus

Semitendinosus

Right leg, posterior view.

Obliques

Rectus abdominis

Sartorius

Gluteus maximus

Tensor faciae latae

Pectoralis major

Deltoid

Triceps brachii

Biceps brachii

Pectineus

Adductor longus

Gracilis

Objectives of exercise
Develop trunk stability. Enhance control of the hip flexors and hip extensors.

Exercise description
- Kneel up straight, and reach both arms out to the side at shoulder height.
- Take one leg out to the side and straighten in line with the body, and place the foot on the mat.
- Lean the body away from this straight leg, and while lifting this straight leg out, place the hand onto the mat under the shoulder; the arm remains straight.
- The raised leg should get to pelvis height. Place the top hand behind the head in this stretched position.
- Return to the start position, and repeat on the opposite side.

Cues to exercise
Lengthening away from the centre.

Breathing pattern
Breathe out when reaching out. Breathe in when lowering the leg.

Checkpoint
- Controlled raised leg, parallel to floor.

Pitfalls
- Losing length through the body.
- Rotating as you raise the leg.
- Losing neutral pelvis.

Muscle focus
Hip abductors. Hip adductors. Shoulder stabilizers. Abdominals.

THE TWIST

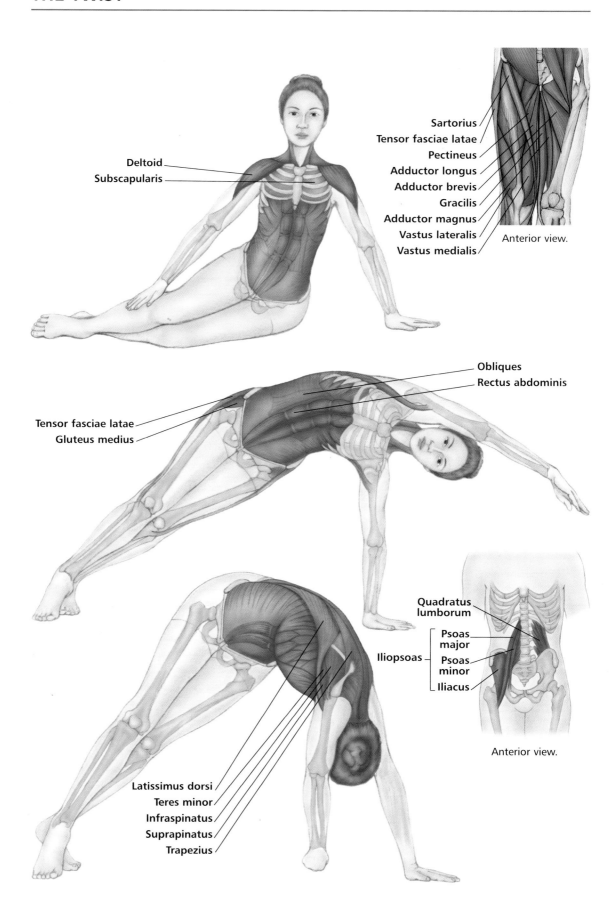

Deltoid
Subscapularis

Sartorius
Tensor fasciae latae
Pectineus
Adductor longus
Adductor brevis
Gracilis
Adductor magnus
Vastus lateralis
Vastus medialis

Anterior view.

Obliques
Rectus abdominis

Tensor fasciae latae
Gluteus medius

Quadratus
lumborum

Iliopsoas

Psoas
major
Psoas
minor
Iliacus

Anterior view.

Latissimus dorsi
Teres minor
Infraspinatus
Suprapinatus
Trapezius

Objectives of exercise

Stretch the side of the body (quadratus lumborum and obliques). Strengthen latissimus dorsi, shoulder stabilizers, gluteals and abdominals.

Exercise description

- Sit on your right hip with your right leg bent, and the foot in line with the pelvis and trunk.
- Cross the left foot over the right ankle, keeping the sole of the foot flat on the mat. Keep the left hip open and externally rotated, and the knee lifted.
- Place the right palm flat on the mat at arms length in line with the pelvis.
- Extend the left arm in a diagonal line and the forearm just in front of the left knee, with the palm facing forward.
- Begin to lift the pelvis and raise the left arm in a circular motion overhead, and simultaneously straighten the legs.
- Rotate the upper trunk to the right so that the chest is facing the mat; this movement helps lift the pelvis further up. Reach through with your arm under your body.
- Return from this rotated position and bring the left arm directly above the left shoulder.
- Return the body to the mat, bending the knees and circling the arm back to the starting position. Repeat on the opposite side.

Cues to exercise

The closer the feet are to the pelvis, the more difficult the stretch is once the body lifts. Use the abdominals to start the movement and the twist of the spine.

Breathing pattern

Breathe in on the way up. Breathe out on the way down.

Checkpoints

- Ensure that the exercise remains smooth. Maintain a smooth arc with your arms and twist through the legs.
- Maintain reach through the arms.
- Control and concentrate on the deep abdominals throughout.
- Maintain alignment of the head and trunk throughout.
- Maintain an open chest throughout.

Pitfalls

- Locking out the elbows; keep them long but slightly bent.
- Loss of control in the supporting scapular.

Muscle focus

Scapular muscles. Adductors. Rotator cuff muscles. Quadratus lumborum. Obliques.

BOOMERANG

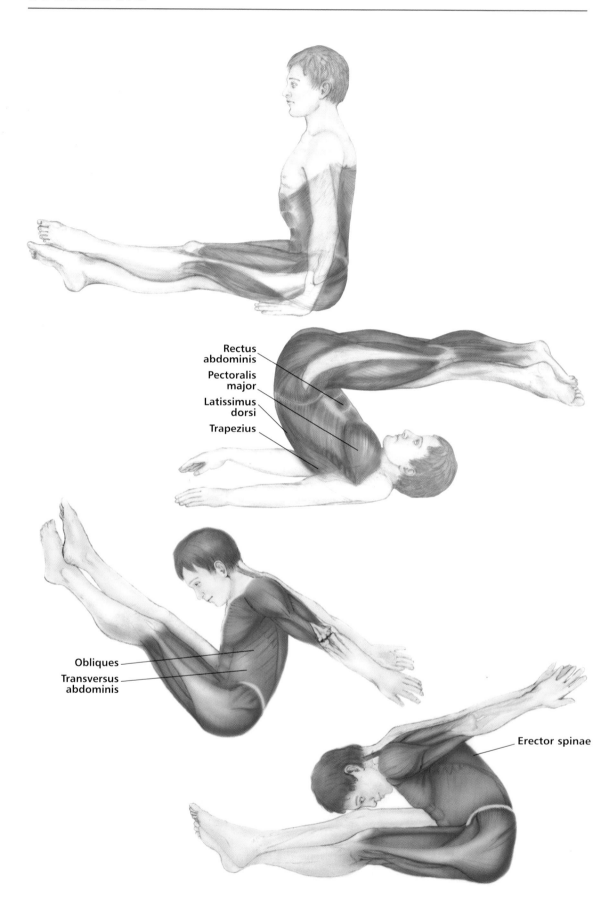

Rectus abdominis

Pectoralis major

Latissimus dorsi

Trapezius

Obliques

Transversus abdominis

Erector spinae

Objectives of exercise

Strengthen the abdominals and back extensors. Enhance hip flexor control. Develop balance through movement.

Exercise description

- Sit upright with your legs straight in front of the body. The legs should be slightly turned out and crossed.
- Keep the arms straight down by the sides of the trunk. Palms flat to the mat, with the fingers pointing forward.
- Lengthen out your hips.
- Press the hands down into the mat and roll the spine backward, lifting the legs to maintain the same degree of hip flexion. Keep rolling through the spine to the tip of the shoulder blades, and keep the legs parallel to (but off) the mat.
- Rapidly uncross and re-cross your legs.
- Maintain straight legs, lift your arms and roll forward.
- During the roll, move your arms out to your sides, around and behind you.
- Clasp your hands and stretch out your arms as far and up as possible.
- Control the movement, stopping the feet just off the ground, and maintain your balance.
- Legs straight, arms stretched out behind you, trunk straight.
- Finish the roll forward, pressing your trunk down onto your legs and raising your arms as high as possible behind you.
- Repeat, re-crossing your legs again as you roll back onto your shoulders.

Cues to exercise

Care with the choreography with the exercise; build the components.

Breathing pattern

Breathe in as you begin to roll back. Breathe out when you have reached the end of your roll and re-crossed your legs. Breathe in when rolling up to the balance point. Breathe out as you press your trunk into your legs.

Checkpoints

- Deep abdominals required throughout.
- Maintain the chin to chest.
- Keep the legs straight throughout.

Pitfalls

- Excessive range of movement made possible through the ribs moving.
- Locking out of the elbows.
- Rolling over too far; take the weight only to the upper back, and not onto either the neck or head.

Muscle focus

Abdominals. Back extensors. Pectorals.

SEAL

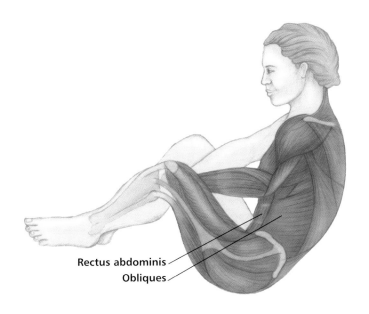

Rectus abdominis
Obliques

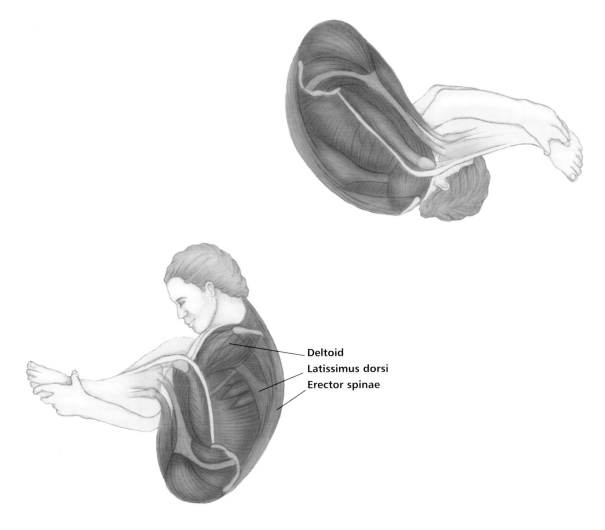

Deltoid
Latissimus dorsi
Erector spinae

Objectives of exercise
Use momentum to stretch the spine. Work the abdominals. Enhance balance and coordination.

Exercise description
- Maintain a strong C-curve of your spine, pressing the soles of your feet together.
- Lift your feet off the mat and control the balance position.
- Open your knees and reach through the space between your knees, bringing your hands outside your ankles and wrapping them around your feet.
- Roll smoothly onto your back. Move your weight from between your shoulders and neck to a balance point, with your toes just off the mat.
- At the balance point, spread your feet apart, and then back together.
- Clapping action.
- Repeat the rolling action.

Cues to exercise
Roll in a straight line.

Breathing pattern
Breathe in on the way up. Breathe out on the way back.

Checkpoints
- Strong deep abdominals.
- Maintain the chin on chest.
- Maintain a smooth motion back and forth.

Pitfalls
- Losing feet and arm position.
- Control through the abdominals.
- Losing the C-shape spine.

Muscle focus
Abdominals. Back extensors.

ROCKING

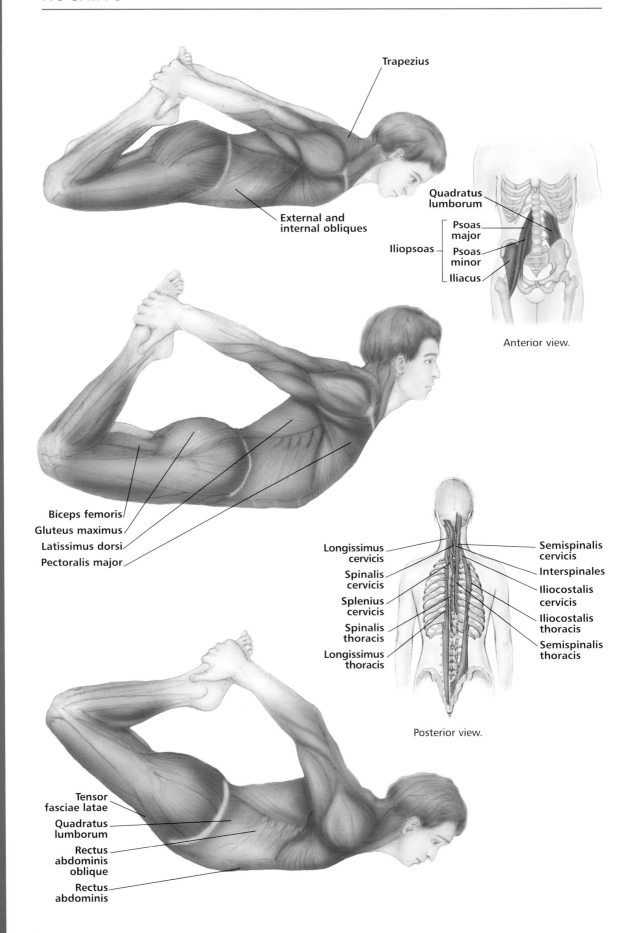

Trapezius

Quadratus lumborum

Iliopsoas
- Psoas major
- Psoas minor
- Iliacus

Anterior view.

External and internal obliques

Biceps femoris
Gluteus maximus
Latissimus dorsi
Pectoralis major

Longissimus cervicis
Spinalis cervicis
Splenius cervicis
Spinalis thoracis
Longissimus thoracis

Semispinalis cervicis
Interspinales
Iliocostalis cervicis
Iliocostalis thoracis
Semispinalis thoracis

Posterior view.

Tensor fasciae latae
Quadratus lumborum
Rectus abdominis oblique
Rectus abdominis

Objectives of exercise

Control rhythm and coordination. Enhance control in spinal extension. Improve hip flexor flexibility.

Exercise description

- Lie on your stomach, bend the knees, and bring the heels toward your bottom.
- Reach the arms behind the body and hold onto the ankles.
- Maintain the legs hip-width apart.
- Press the ankles into the hands, lift and pull the spine into extension off the mat.
- Rock forward on the chest bone, pulling the ankles up behind the bottom.

Cues to exercise

The back is like the rim of a wheel. Develop a rhythm in the movement.

Breathing pattern

Breathe out on the way forward. Breathe in, with force, on the lift and pulling to give momentum.

Checkpoints

- Strong deep abdominals.
- Use leg and back muscles to pull your feet toward the mat.
- Keep the head drawn back.
- Maintain an even arch.
- Relax a tight chest.

Muscle focus

Back extensors. Pectorals. Abdominals.

CONTROL AND BALANCE

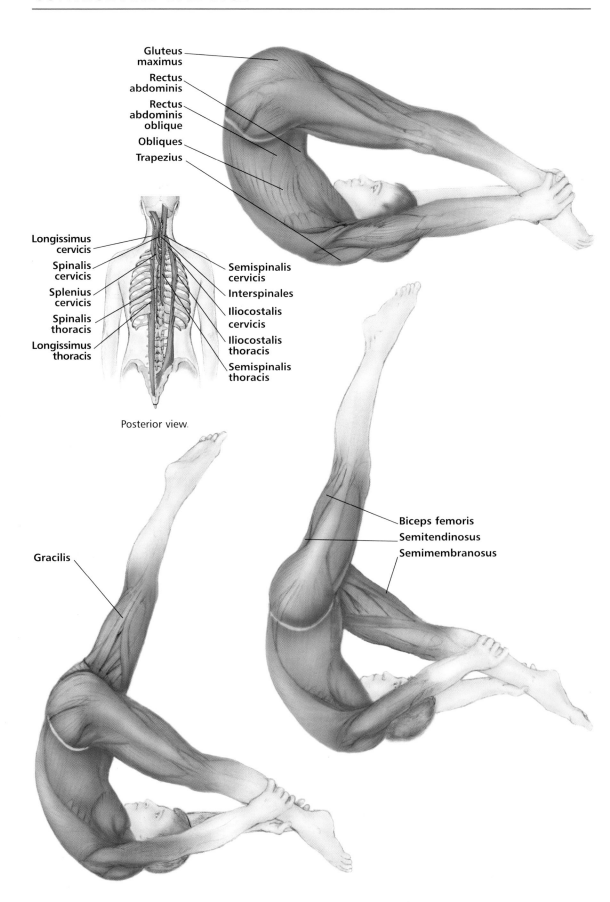

Gluteus maximus

Rectus abdominis

Rectus abdominis oblique

Obliques

Trapezius

Longissimus cervicis

Spinalis cervicis

Splenius cervicis

Spinalis thoracis

Longissimus thoracis

Semispinalis cervicis

Interspinales

Iliocostalis cervicis

Iliocostalis thoracis

Semispinalis thoracis

Posterior view.

Gracilis

Biceps femoris

Semitendinosus

Semimembranosus

Objectives of exercise

Teach balance and coordination. Improve hip flexor flexibility. Enhance core strength.

Exercise description

- Lie on your back, with the arms shoulder-width apart next to your head, and the legs straight and together.
- Keeping the legs straight, swing them up off the mat and over your head. The toes need to touch the floor beyond your head.
- Take hold of one ankle with both hands.
- Reach up with the opposite leg, stretching out of your hip, while holding the ankle and keeping the opposite foot on or near to the floor.
- Reverse the hold on your ankle smoothly as it approaches the mat. Reach for the ceiling with the toes on the opposite foot.

Cues to exercise

Lift the legs and pelvis away from the spine to enhance control. Leg change over at 45 degrees to the mat.

Breathing pattern

Breathe in as one leg reaches up. Breathe out as you bring it down and the other reaches up.

Checkpoints

- Maintain straight legs.
- Strong deep abdominal contraction.

Pitfalls

- Forcing your breathing; keep natural rhythm with the leg movement.
- Touching the mat with your foot as you draw it over your head.
- Rolling too far. Maintain your weight across the upper back, not the head and neck.

Muscle focus

Abdominals. Hip extensors. Back extensors.

PUSH-UP

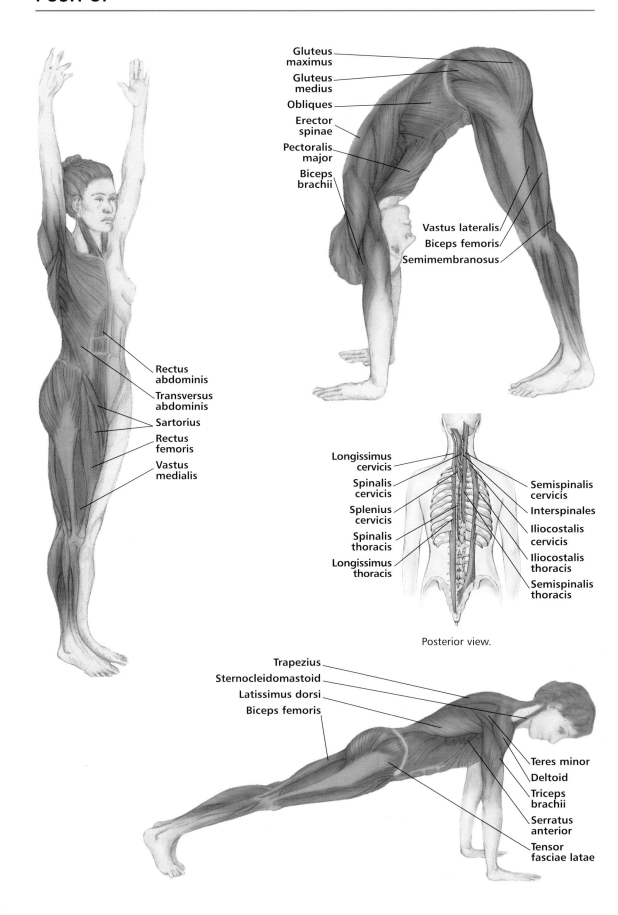

Gluteus maximus
Gluteus medius
Obliques
Erector spinae
Pectoralis major
Biceps brachii

Vastus lateralis
Biceps femoris
Semimembranosus

Rectus abdominis
Transversus abdominis
Sartorius
Rectus femoris
Vastus medialis

Longissimus cervicis
Spinalis cervicis
Splenius cervicis
Spinalis thoracis
Longissimus thoracis

Semispinalis cervicis
Interspinales
Iliocostalis cervicis
Iliocostalis thoracis
Semispinalis thoracis

Posterior view.

Trapezius
Sternocleidomastoid
Latissimus dorsi
Biceps femoris

Teres minor
Deltoid
Triceps brachii
Serratus anterior
Tensor fasciae latae

Objectives of exercise

Strengthen elbow extensors and the pectoralis muscle group. Enhance trunk control. Enhance movement sequencing.

Exercise description

- Standing in a Pilates stance, raise the arms directly above the head, shoulder-width apart, and the palms facing forward.
- Lower the arms, initiating with a nod of the neck, roll the spine down sequentially until the hands reach the mat.
- Begin to walk the hands out in front of the legs, allowing your heels to lift until you are in a push-up position.
- Place the hands directly under the shoulders with the spine and pelvis in neutral, and the trunk forming a straight line.
- Bend the elbows, keeping the elbows close in toward the trunk. Lower the body to just above the floor.
- Push out through the elbows, pressing the body back to the plank position. Repeat.
- Reverse walk the hands back toward your feet, creating a V-shape from the hips. When your hands are close to your feet, curl up through the body, and return to standing.

Cues to exercise

Maintain contraction of the abdominals and gluteals (this avoids a sagging posture). Keep your head in line with the body.

Breathing pattern

Breathe in when walking your hands down your legs. Breathe out when walking your hands along the mat. Breathe in on the push-up 'down' movement. Breathe out on the way up. Breathe in when walking back toward your feet. Breathe out when curling up to standing.

Checkpoints

- Strong abdominals throughout.
- Maintain a straight line on the walk out.
- Maintain a neutral spine in plank position.

Pitfalls

- Allowing the push-up action to sag through the trunk.
- Hunching up your shoulders.
- Elbows too close to your body during the press down action; maintain a soft elbow (don't lock out).

Muscle focus

Abdominals. Quadriceps. Hip flexors. Gluteals. Shoulder stabilizers. Pectorals. Triceps brachii. Hamstrings. Back extensors.

MERMAID

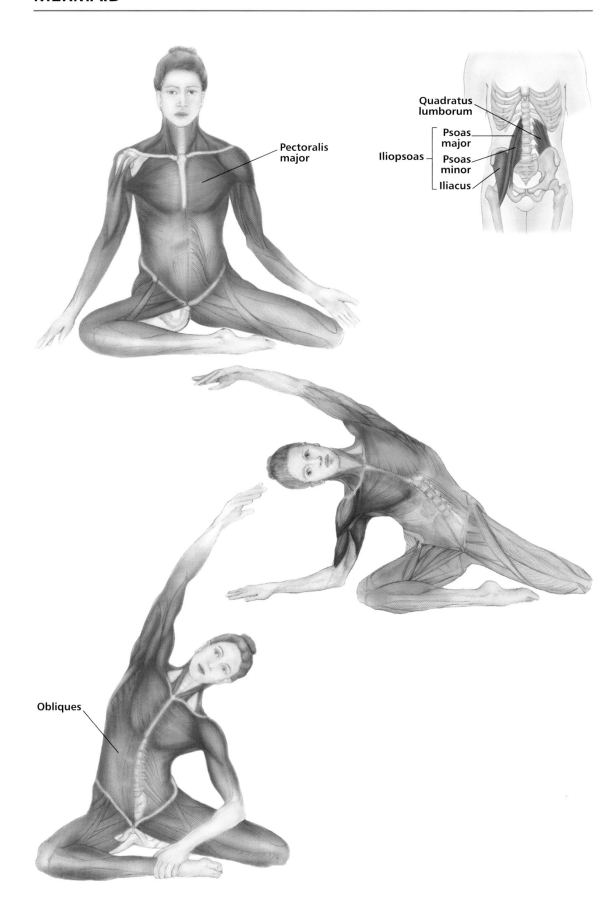

Pectoralis major

Quadratus lumborum

Iliopsoas

Psoas major

Psoas minor

Iliacus

Obliques

Objectives of exercise
Deep muscle stretch in the lateral trunk flexors. Enhance mobility throughout the spine.

Exercise description
• Sit, with the right knee in front, bent and externally rotated, and the back knee bent and internally rotated.
• Place one hand onto the floor as you side bend your trunk, reaching up and over with the opposite arm.
• Lift back up to sitting, reaching up and over the opposite side, side-bending the trunk.

Cues to exercise
Bring weight forward to the front hip, with reduced compression on the back knee.

Breathing pattern
Breathe in to prepare. Breathe out as you stretch out.

Checkpoints
• Keep the reaching arm in line with your ear and neck.
• Maintain length in the sides; try not to collapse into the side bend.
• Remain square in the front and ribs.

Pitfalls
• Arching the back.

Muscle focus
Abdominal obliques. Quadratus lumborum. Latissimus dorsi. Pectorals.

SPINE CURLS

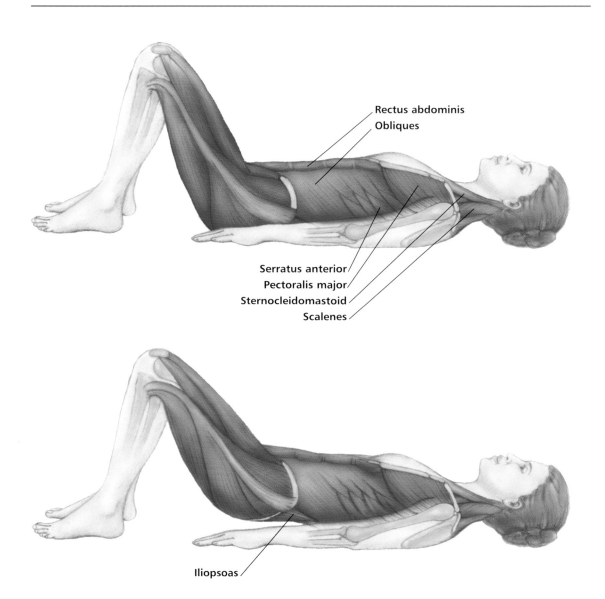

Rectus abdominis
Obliques

Serratus anterior
Pectoralis major
Sternocleidomastoid
Scalenes

Iliopsoas

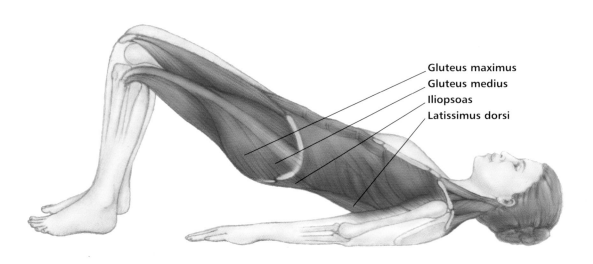

Gluteus maximus
Gluteus medius
Iliopsoas
Latissimus dorsi

Not a classic Pilates mat exercise, but a good exercise for spinal alignment.

Objectives of exercise
Enhance the segmental control in the lumbar spine. Lengthen the latissimus dorsi muscle.

Exercise description
- Lie on your back with your knees bent and feet on the floor, hip-width apart. Arms placed at your side on the floor.
- Engage your lower abdominal muscles, and slowly curl from your base of the spine. Allow each spinal segment to curl and lift off the floor in a sequence.
- Rise to a point whereby you balance on your shoulder blades.
- Hold the end position, and then reverse the movement to return to the start position.

Cue to exercise
Curl the spine like a wheel.

Breathing pattern
Breathe in to prepare. Breathe out as you curl up your spine. Breathe in as you hold the raised position.

Checkpoints
- Maintain equal weight on your feet.
- Maintain the curl of the spine throughout the movement.
- Maintain a level pelvis; take care not to drop on one side whilst raising through the curl.

Pitfalls
- Rising onto your shoulder blades; to a point along the thoracic spine.
- Rushing the curl action at the start of the movement; work segmentally in a sequence.

Muscle focus
Abdominals. Latissimus dorsi. Psoas. Gluteals. Erector spinae. Hamstrings.

Glossary of Terms

Agonist.	See prime mover.
Antagonist.	A muscle on the opposite side of a joint to the prime mover, and which must relax to allow the prime mover to contract.
Concentric contraction.	The muscle attachments move closer together, causing movement at the joint.
Eccentric contraction.	The muscle fibres 'pay out' in a controlled manner to slow down movements which gravity, if unchecked, would otherwise cause to be too rapid.
Fixator.	A synergist is more specifically referred to as a fixator (or stabilizer) when it immobilizes the bone of the prime mover's origin, thus providing a stable base for the action of the prime mover.
Flat back posture.	Reduced lumbar curve.
Intra-abdominal pressure.	Pressure created in the trunk, in the closed cylinder of the diaphragm, pelvic floor and abdominal wall.
Isometric contraction.	An isometric contraction occurs when a muscle increases its tension, but the length of the muscle is not altered.
Isotonic contraction.	Contraction of a muscle that results in the muscle creating movement.
Kyphosis.	Excessive curvature in the thoracic region of the spine.
Lordosis.	Excessive curvature in the lumbar region of the spine.
Mobilizer.	A muscle responsible for movement.
Muscle slings.	Coupling mechanism between the core areas, which allows for the transfer of force of movement between them.
Neutralizer.	See synergist.

Neutral spine.	Defined as the position of the anterior superior iliac spine (ASIS) and the pubic symphysis in neutral when the ASIS lies parallel in the transverse plane. Natural curves of the spine.
Prime mover.	A muscle that contracts to produce a specified movement.
Proprioception.	Awareness of the joint–body position, generated by sensory feedback.
Stabilizer.	See fixator.
Sway back posture.	Indicated by the hips pushed forward and anterior tilt of the pelvis.
Synergist.	A muscle which prevents any unwanted movements that might occur as the prime mover contracts.
Thoraco-lumbar fascia.	Thick connective tissue sheath, which helps to stabilize the trunk and pelvis.
Trunk stability.	The ability to maintain the trunk position while working the limbs.

Anatomical Directions

Abduction.	A movement away from the midline (or to return from adduction).
Adduction.	A movement toward the midline (or to return from abduction).
Anatomical position.	The body is upright with the arms and hands turned forward.
Anterior.	Towards the front of the body (as opposed to posterior).
Caudal.	Directed toward the tail; inferior.
Circumduction.	Movement in which the distal end of a bone moves in a circle, while the proximal end remains stable.
Contralateral.	On the opposite side.
Coronal plane.	A vertical plane at right angles to the sagittal plane that divides the body into anterior and posterior portions.
Deep.	Away from the surface (as opposed to superficial).
Depression.	Movement of an elevated part of the body downwards to its original position.
Distal.	Away from the point of origin of a structure (as opposed to proximal).
Dorsal.	Relating to the back or posterior portion (as opposed to ventral).
Elevation.	Movement of a part of the body upwards along the frontal plane.
Eversion.	To turn the sole of the foot outward.
Extension.	A movement at a joint resulting in separation of two ventral surfaces (as opposed to flexion).
Flexion.	A movement at a joint resulting in approximation of two ventral surfaces (as opposed to extension).
Frontal plane.	See coronal plane.
Horizontal plane.	A transverse plane at right angle to the long axis of the body.
Inferior.	Below or furthest away from the head.
Inversion.	To turn the sole of the foot inward.

Lateral.	Located away from the midline opposite to medial).
Medial.	Situated close to or at the midline of the body or organ (opposite to lateral).
Median.	Centrally located, situated in the middle of the body.
Opposition.	A movement specific to the saddle joint of the thumb that enables you to touch your thumb to the tips of the fingers of the same hand.
Palmar.	Anterior surface of the hand.
Plantar.	The sole of the foot.
Posterior.	Relating to the back or the dorsal aspect of the body (opposite to anterior).
Pronation.	To turn the palm of the hand down to face the floor, or away from the anatomical and foetal positions.
Prone.	Position of the body in which the ventral surface faces down (as opposed to supine).
Protraction.	Movement forwards in the transverse plane.
Proximal.	Closer to the centre of the body or to the point of attachment of a limb.
Retraction.	Movement backwards in the transverse plane.
Rotation.	Move around a fixed axis.
Sagittal plane.	A vertical plane extending in an antero-posterior direction dividing the body into right and left parts.
Superficial.	On or near the surface (as opposed to deep).
Superior.	Above or closest to the head.
Supination.	To turn the palm of the hand up to face the ceiling, or toward the anatomical and foetal positions.
Supine.	Position of the body in which the ventral surface faces up (as opposed to prone).
Transverse plane.	Horizontal cross-section, dividing the body into upper and lower sections, and lies at right angles to the other two planes.
Ventral.	Refers to the anterior part of the body (as opposed to dorsal).

Muscle Groups

Deep Neck Flexors
Longus Colli
Longus Capitis

Scalenes
Scalenus Anterior
Scalenus Medius
Scalenus Posterior

Erector Spinae
Iliocostalis Cervicis, Thoracis, Lumborum
Longissimus Capitis, Cervicis, Thoracis
Spinalis Cervicis, Thoracis

Scapular Stabilizers
Lower Trapezius
Serratus Anterior
Latissimus Dorsi

Rotator Cuff
Supraspinatus
Infraspinatus
Teres Minor
Subscapularis

**Abdominals
(Anterior Abdominal Wall)**
Obliques
Transversus Abdominis
Rectus Abdominis

**Abdominals
(Posterior Abdominal Wall)**
Quadratus Lumborum
Psoas Major
Iliacus

Gluteals
Gluteus Maximus
Gluteus Minimus
Gluteus Medius

Medial Hip Rotators
Gluteus Medius
Gluteus Minimus
Tensor Fasciae Latae
Adductor Magnus (part)
Pectineus (when leg abducted)

Deep Lateral Hip Rotators
Obturator Internus
Gemellus Superior
Gemellus Inferior
Quadratus Femoris

Hamstrings
Biceps Femoris
Semitendinosus
Semimembranosus

Adductors
Adductor Magnus
Adductor Brevis
Adductor Longus

Quadriceps
Rectus Femoris
Vastus Lateralis
Vastus Medialis
Vastus Intermedius

Main Muscles Involved in Movement

Atlanto-occipital and Atlanto-axial Joints

Flexion
Longus Capitis; Rectus Capitis Anterior; Sternocleidomastoideus (anterior fibres)

Extension
Semispinalis Capitis; Splenius Capitis; Rectus Capitis Posterior Major; Rectus Capitis Posterior Minor; Obliquus Capitis Superior; Longissimus Capitis; Trapezius; Sternocleidomastoideus (posterior fibres)

Rotation and Lateral Flexion
Sternocleidomastoideus; Obliquus Capitis Inferior; Obliquus Capitis Superior; Rectus Capitis Lateralis; Longissimus Capitis; Splenius Capitis

Intervertebral Joints

Cervical Region

Flexion
Longus Colli; Longus Capitis; Sternocleidomastoideus

Extension
Longissimus Cervicis; Longissimus Capitis; Splenius Capitis; Splenius Cervicis; Semispinalis Cervicis; Semispinalis Capitis; Trapezius; Interspinales; Iliocostalis Cervicis

Rotation and Lateral Flexion
Longissimus Cervicis; Longissimus Capitis; Splenius Capitis; Splenius Cervicis; Multifidis; Longus Colli; Scalenus Anterior; Scalenus Medius; Scalenus Posterior; Sternocleidomastoideus; Levator Scapulae; Iliocostalis Cervicis; Intertransversarii

Thoracic and/or Lumbar Regions

Flexion
Obliques; Transversus Abdominis; Rectus Abdominis

Extension
Erector Spinae; Quadratus Lumborum; Trapezius

Rotation and Lateral Flexion
Iliocostalis Lumborum; Iliocostalis Thoracis; Multifidis; Rotatores; Intertransversarii; Quadratus Lumborum; Psoas Major; Obliques; Transversus Abdominis; Rectus Abdominis

Shoulder Girdle

Elevation
Trapezius (upper fibres); Levator Scapulae; Rhomboideus Minor; Rhomboideus Major; Sternocleidomastoideus

Depression
Trapezius (lower fibres); Pectoralis Minor; Pectoralis Major (sternocostal portion); Latissimus Dorsi

Protraction
Serratus Anterior; Pectoralis Minor; Pectoralis Major

Retraction
Trapezius (middle fibres); Rhomboideus Minor; Rhomboideus Major; Latissimus Dorsi

Lateral Displacement of Inferior Angle of Scapula
Serratus Anterior; Trapezius (upper and lower fibres)

Medial Displacement of Inferior Angle of Scapula
Pectoralis Minor; Rhomboideus Minor; Rhomboideus Major; Latissimus Dorsi

Shoulder Joint

Flexion
Deltoideus (anterior portion); Pectoralis Major (clavicular portion: sternocostal portion flexes the extended humerus as far as the position of rest); Biceps Brachii; Coracobrachialis

Extension
Deltoideus (posterior portion); Teres Major (of flexed humerus); Latissimus Dorsi (of flexed humerus); Pectoralis Major (sternocostal portion of flexed humerus); Triceps Brachii (long head to position of rest)

Abduction
Deltoideus (middle portion); Supraspinatus; Biceps Brachii (long head)

Adduction
Pectoralis Major; Teres Major; Latissimus Dorsi; Triceps Brachii (long head); Coracobrachialis

Lateral Rotation
Deltoideus (posterior portion); Infraspinatus; Teres Minor

Medial Rotation
Pectoralis Major; Teres Major; Latissimus Dorsi; Deltoideus (anterior portion); Subscapularis

Horizontal Flexion
Deltoideus (anterior portion); Pectoralis Major; Subscapularis

Horizontal Extension
Deltoideus (posterior portion); Infraspinatus

Elbow Joint

Flexion
Brachialis; Biceps Brachii;
Brachioradialis; Extensor Carpi
Radialis Longus; Pronator Teres;
Flexor Carpi Radialis

Extension
Triceps Brachii; Anconeus

Radio-ulnar Joint

Supination
Supinator; Biceps Brachii; Extensor
Pollicis Longus

Pronation
Pronator Quadratus; Pronator Teres;
Flexor Carpi Radialis

Radiocarpal and Midcarpal Joints

Flexion
Flexor Carpi Radialis; Flexor Carpi
Ulnaris; Palmaris Longus; Flexor
Digitorum Superficialis; Flexor
Digitorum Profundus; Flexor Pollicis
Longus; Abductor Pollicis Longus;
Extensor Pollicis Brevis

Extension
Extensor Carpi Radialis Brevis;
Extensor Carpi Radialis Longus;
Extensor Carpi Ulnaris; Extensor
Digitorum; Extensor Indicis; Extensor
Pollicis Longus; Extensor Digiti
Minimi

Abduction
Extensor Carpi Radialis Brevis;
Extensor Carpi Radialis Longus;
Flexor Carpi Radialis; Abductor
Pollicis Longus; Extensor Pollicis
Longus; Extensor Pollicis Brevis

Adduction
Flexor Carpi Ulnaris; Extensor Carpi
Ulnaris

Metacarpophalangeal Joints of the Fingers

Flexion
Flexor Digitorum Profundus; Flexor Digitorum Superficialis; Lumbricales; Interossei; Flexor Digiti Minimi; Abductor Digiti Minimi; Palmaris Longus (through palmar aponeurosis)

Extension
Extensor Digitorum; Extensor Indicis; Extensor Digiti Minimi

Abduction and Adduction
Interossei; Abductor Digiti Minimi; Lumbricales (may assist in radial deviation); Extensor Digitorum (abducts by hyperextending; tendon to index radially deviates); Flexor Digitorum Profundus (adducts by flexing); Flexor Digitorum Superficialis (adducts by flexing)

Rotation
Lumbricales; Interossei (movement slight except index; only effective when phalanx is flexed); Opponens Digiti Minimi (rotates little finger at carpometacarpal joint)

Hip Joint

Flexion
Iliopsoas; Rectus Femoris; Tensor Fasciae Latae; Sartorius; Adductor Brevis; Adductor Longus; Pectineus

Extension
Gluteus Maximus; Semitendinosus; Semimembranosus; Biceps Femoris (long head); Adductor Magnus (ischial fibres)

Abduction
Gluteus Medius; Gluteus Minimus; Tensor Fasciae Latae; Obturator Internus (in flexion); Piriformis (in flexion)

Adduction
Adductor Magnus; Adductor Brevis; Adductor Longus; Pectineus; Gracilis; Gluteus Maximus (lower fibres); Quadratus Femoris

Lateral Rotation
Gluteus Maximus; Obturator Internus; Gemelli; Obturator Externus; Quadratus Femoris; Piriformis; Sartorius; Adductor Magnus; Adductor Brevis; Adductor Longus

Medial Rotation
Iliopsoas (in initial stage of flexion); Tensor Fasciae Latae; Gluteus Medius (anterior fibres); Gluteus Minimus (anterior fibres)

Knee Joint

Flexion
Semitendinosus; Semimembranosus;
Biceps Femoris; Gastrocnemius;
Plantaris; Sartorius; Gracilis;
Popliteus

Extension
Quadratus Femoris

Medial Rotation of Tibia on Femur
Popliteus; Semitendinosus;
Semimembranosus; Sartorius; Gracilis

Lateral Rotation of Tibia on Femur
Biceps Femoris

Ankle Joint

Dorsiflexion
Tibialis Anterior, Extensor Hallucis
Longus; Extensor Digitorum Longus;
Fibularis (Peroneus) Tertius

Plantar Flexion
Gastrocnemius; Plantaris; Soleus;
Tibialis Posterior; Flexor Hallucis
Longus; Flexor Digitorum Longus;
Fibularis (Peroneus) Longus; Fibularis
(Peroneus) Brevis

Intertarsal Joints

Inversion
Tibialis Anterior; Tibialis Posterior

Eversion
Fibularis (Peroneus) Tertius; Fibularis
(Peroneus) Longus; Fibularis
(Peroneus) Brevis

Other Movements
Sliding movements which allow some
dorsiflexion, plantar flexion,
abduction and adduction, are
produced by the muscles acting on
the toes. Tibialis Anterior, Tibialis
Posterior, and Fibularis (Peroneus)
Tertius are also involved.

Resources

Anderson, D. M. (chief Lexicographer): 2003. *Dorland's Illustrated Medical Dictionary, 30th edition.* Saunders, an imprint of Elsevier, Philadelphia

Bass, M., Robinson, L. & Thomson, G.: 2005. *The Complete Classic Pilates Method: Centre Yourself With This Step-by-step Approach to Joseph Pilates' Original Matwork Programme.* Macmillan, London

Elphinston, J.: 2008: *Stability, Sport and Performance Movement: Great Technique Without Injury.* Lotus Publishing, Chichester / North Atlantic Books, Berkeley

Friedman, P. & Eisen, G.: 2004. *The Pilates Method of Physical and Mental Conditioning.* Penguin, London

Gallagher, S. P.: 2000. *Joseph H. Pilates Archive Collection: The Photographs, Writings and Designs.* Bainbridge Books.

Kendall, F. P., and McCreary, E. K.: 1983. *Muscles, Testing & Function, 3rd edition.* Williams & Wilkins, Baltimore

Herman, E.: 2007. *Ellie Herman's Pilates Mat.* Ellie Herman Books, Brooklyn

Isacowitz, R.: 2006. *Pilates.* Human Kinetics, Champaign

Jarmey, C.: 2008. *The Concise Book of Muscles, 2nd edition.* Lotus Publishing, Chichester / North Atlantic Books, Berkeley

Jarmey, C.: 2006. *The Concise Book of the Moving Body.* Lotus Publishing, Chichester / North Atlantic Books, Berkeley

Latey, P.: 2001. *Modern Pilates: The Step by Step, at Home Guide to a Stronger Body.* Allen & Unwin, London

Lyon, D.: 2006. *The Complete Book of Pilates For Men.* Harper Collins, London

Massey, P.: 2004. *Sports Pilates: How to Prevent and Overcome Injuries.* Cico Books, London

Myers, T. W.: 2001. *Anatomy Trains.* Elsevier, Edinburgh

Norris, C.M.: 1998. *Sports Injuries: Diagnosis and Management.* Butterworth Heinemann, Oxford, UK

Norris, C. M.: 2000. *Back Stability.* Human Kinetics, Champaign

Pilates, J. H.: 1934. *Your Health: A Corrective System of Exercising That Revolutionizes the Entire Field of Physical Education.*

Pilates, J. H. & Miller, W. J.: 1945. *Return to Life through Controlology and Your Health.*

Richardson, C., Jull, G., Hodges, P. & Hides, J.: 1998. *Therapeutic Exercise for Spinal Segmental Stabilisation in Low Back Pain.* Churchill Livingstone, Edinburgh

Romanes, G. J. (editor): 1972. *Cunningham's Textbook of Anatomy, 11th edition.* Oxford University Press, London

Siler, B.: 2000. *The Pilates Body.* Michael Joseph, London

Walker, B.E.: 2007. *The Anatomy of Stretching.* Lotus Publishing, Chichester/ North Atlantic Books, Berkeley

Index of Pilates Exercises

Gloss Laminated Wall Charts

Using drawings taken from the best-selling *The Anatomy of Stretching*, these beautifully illustrated wall charts show exactly what is happening during a stretch. Each of the 16 key stretches illustrates the primary and secondary muscles worked, showing how to perform each stretch and highlight sports injuries for which each stretch will be beneficial.

Aimed at fitness professionals, physical therapists, sports scientists, or anyone involved in sport, these charts will help explain what is happening during a stretch, how the stretch can assist in recovery from injury, and add colour to any gym or treatment room wall.

PRICE: **£10.99** plus VAT
FORMAT: 995mm x 740mm

Upper Body Stretches
(ISBN 978 1 905367 14 6)

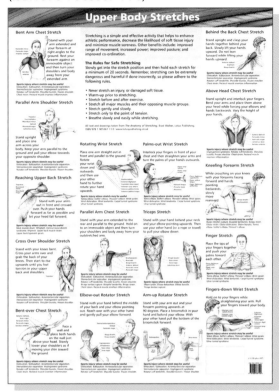

Lower Body Stretches
(ISBN 978 1 905367 15 3)

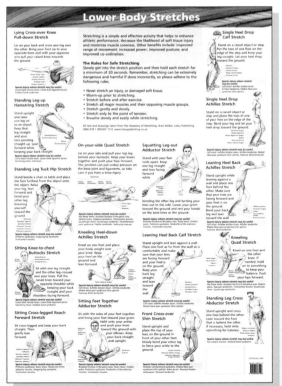

Neck, Back and Core Stretches
(ISBN 978 1 905367 16 0)

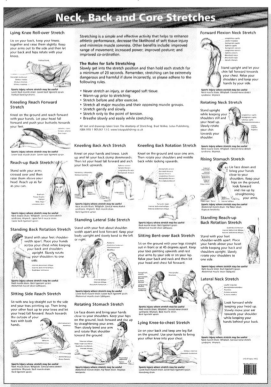

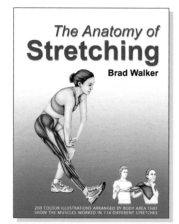

The Anatomy of Stretching — Brad Walker

978 1 905367 03 0 (UK)/978 1 55643 596 (US); **£14.99/$24.95**;
176 pages; 265 mm x 194 mm; 320 colour illustrations; paperback

Books on stretching are common, but *The Anatomy of Stretching* takes a more fundamental approach than the others, taking the reader inside the body to show exactly what is happening during a stretch. At the heart of the book are 300 full-colour illustrations that show the primary and secondary muscles worked in 114 key stretches arranged by body area. Author Brad Walker brings years of expertise – he works with elite-level and world-champion athletes, and lectures on injury prevention – to this how-to guide. He looks at stretching from every angle, including physiology and flexibility; the benefits of stretching; the different types of stretching; rules for safe stretching; and how to stretch properly. Aimed at fitness enthusiasts of any level, as well as at fitness pros, *The Anatomy of Stretching* also focuses on which stretches are useful for the alleviation or rehabilitation of specific sports injuries.

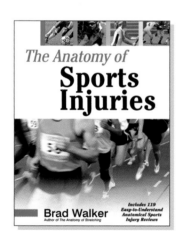

The Anatomy of Sports Injuries — Brad Walker

978 1 905367 06 1 (UK)/ 978 1 55643 666 6 (US); **£16.99/$29.95**;
256 pages; 265 mm x 194 mm; 250 colour / black and white illustrations; paperback

The Anatomy of Sports Injuries takes you inside the body to show exactly what is happening when a sports injury occurs. At the heart of *The Anatomy of Sports Injuries* are 300 full-colour illustrations that show the sports injury in detail, along with 200 line drawings of simple stretching, strengthening, and rehabilitation exercises that the reader can use to speed up the recovery process. *The Anatomy of Sports Injuries* is for every sports player or fitness enthusiast who has been injured and would like to know what the injury involves, how to rehabilitate the area, and how to prevent complications or injury in the future. This book is the perfect partner for Brad's other book, *The Anatomy of Stretching*.

Brad Walker, B.Sc. Health Sciences, is a prominent Australian sports trainer with more than 20 years experience in the health and fitness industry. He graduated from the University of New England, and has postgraduate accreditations in athletics, swimming, and triathlon coaching.

Order from: www.lotuspublishing.co.uk or www.northatlanticbooks.com